COLOUR GUIDE
Surgical Signs

Bruce Campbell MS FRCP FRCS

Consultant Surgeon, Royal Devon and Exeter Hospital, Exeter, UK

Martin Cooper MS FRCS

Consultant Surgeon, Royal Devon and Exeter Hospital, Exeter, UK

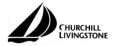

CHURCHILL
LIVINGSTONE

EDINBURGH LONDON MADRID MELBOURNE NEW YORK AND TOKYO 1994

Acknowledgments

We would like to thank the following colleagues who have kindly provided illustrations: Dr R. S. Amin, Mr A. V. Babajews, Mr R. N. Baird, Mr P. Beasley, Professor J. R. Farndon, Dr C. Hamilton-Wood, Professor P. J. Morris, Dr G. D. Morrison, Mr R. D. Pocock, Mr P. R. W. Stanley and Dr A. P. Warin. We also thank the Medical Photogrpahy Departments of the Royal Devon and Exeter Hospital, Bristol Royal Infirmary and John Radcliffe Hospital, Oxford.

Exeter   B. C.
1994   M. C.

Contents

1 / **Skin**

Benign lumps

Sebaceous cyst

Sebaceous cysts are very common. They are trichilemmal or epidermoid cysts arising from skin adnexae, so they are *within* the skin (Fig. 1). They are usually firm and nonfluctuant (because their contents is semi-solid), tense, and may be small. When large they can sometimes be indented. Infection is a common complication and produces fibrosis and scarring, making them difficult to remove.

Neurofibroma

Neurofibromata are rather uncommon. A true neurofibroma arises within a nerve while neurilemmomas arise from the nerve sheath. Both are mobile from side to side across the axis of the nerve, but not longitudinally. Pressure sometimes gives pain or paraesthesiae in the nerve distribution. Neurofibromata can form on the cut ends of nerves and give rise to pain (for example after amputation). Multiple neurofibromatosis (von Recklinghausen's disease, Fig. 2) includes plexiform neurofibromata, which have folds of exuberant skin overlying them.

Seborrhoeic wart (or keratosis)

These benign basal cell papillomata are common in the elderly. They occur most often on the face and trunk (Fig. 3). Usually round, they have a brownish uneven greasy surface. They are not caused by viral infection.

Keloid

Excessive collagen formation in the dermis after surgery or trauma produces a scar which is thickened and raised, and often darker than normal skin (Fig. 4). Keloids are common in Negroes and typical after ear piercing.

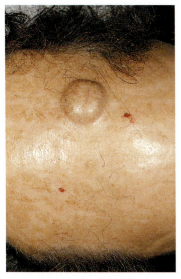

Fig. 1 Sebaceous cyst on scalp.

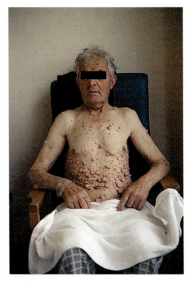

Fig. 2 Multiple neurofibromata.

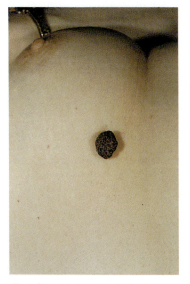

Fig. 3 Seborrhoeic wart on chest.

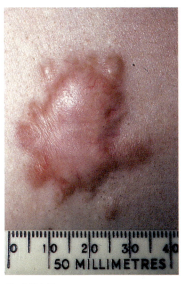

Fig. 4 Keloid scar.

Benign lumps (contd)

Lipoma   Lipomata are very common. These benign tumours of fat usually lie subcutaneously and are freely mobile (Fig. 5). Larger lipomata are soft and sometimes obviously lobulated. Small lipomata are often firmer. Over the scalp and forehead lipomata often lie beneath the epicranial aponeurosis (subfascial lipoma). Lipomata within muscle present as deep-seated swellings. In multiple lipomatosis (Dercum's disease) the lipomata are firm and often tender.

Ganglion   Ganglia are common. They arise from joint capsules or tendon sheaths. A ganglion presents as a well-defined, rounded non-tender lump and consists of a 'cyst' containing gelatinous fluid. They are commonest about the wrist, but also occur around the ankle and foot, the knee, the palm and the fingers (Fig. 6).

Strawberry naevus   These cavernous haemangiomata affect young children. They usually appear soon after birth and enlarge for several months, varying in eventual size from a few millimetres to several centimetres in diameter. Strawberry naevi are raised and deep red in colour (Fig. 7), but become paler and gradually disappear during childhood. This contrasts with the capillary haemangioma (port wine stain) which is present at birth and permanent.

Benign mole   Moles are very common. Most people have several. These naevi may be present at birth or appear in childhood or puberty. The degree of pigmentation varies (Fig. 8), as does the size and morphology. Flat moles are common on the palms and soles. Raised moles elsewhere often bear hairs.

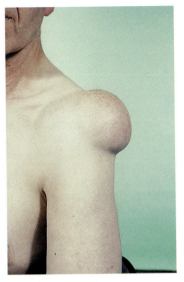

Fig. 5 Lipoma on shoulder.

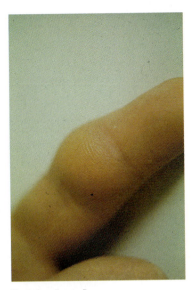

Fig. 6 Ganglion on finger.

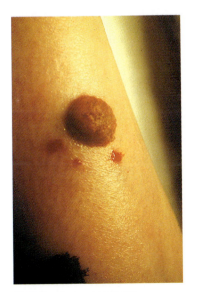

Fig. 7 Strawberry naevus on arm.

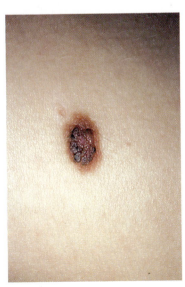

Fig. 8 Benign naevus: this example shows differential pigmentation.

Benign conditions

Hydradenitis suppurativa

This is chronic inflammation of the apocrine sweat glands, which may occur in the axilla (Fig. 9) or in the perineum. Discharging sinuses result, with intermittent abscess formation. Treatment is difficult—drainage, excision, and even skin grafting seldom provide a long-term cure.

Pyogenic granuloma

Lesions occur most commonly on the lips or fingers (Fig. 10). This lesion is dull red, firm, and rapidly growing to a size of up to 2 cm. It is occasionally painful and may bleed. Despite the name there is no definite evidence of an infective cause, and histology shows masses of capillaries without epithelium in an oedematous matrix. Treatment is excision which is curative and allows the diagnosis to be confirmed.

Keratoacanthoma

A dome-shaped reddish lesion grows rapidly over several weeks and then ulcerates centrally. The central keratin plug detaches to leave a crater and if left untreated the lesion regresses completely over a few months. Lesions are commonest on the face, particularly around the lips (Fig. 11) in people aged 50–70 years. The main importance of keratoacanthoma is differential diagnosis from squamous or basal cell carcinoma, and biopsy followed by curettage and cautery is generally recommended. Larger lesions can be treated by radiotherapy.

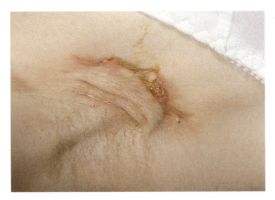

Fig. 9 Hydradenitis of axilla.

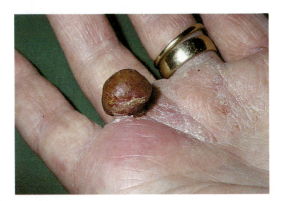

Fig. 10 Pyogenic granuloma of hand.

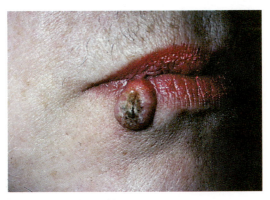

Fig. 11 Keratoacanthoma of lip.

Malignancy

Basal cell carcinoma

These common malignant tumours of skin invade locally (rodent ulcer) but do not metastasize. Commonest on the face (Fig. 12), they usually present as a small ulcer with a raised pearly telangiectatic edge. In the cystic type there is no central ulceration. Rarely they are pigmented resembling a melanoma. Treatment is by excision, curettage and cautery, or by local radiotherapy.

Squamous cell carcinoma

Initially nodular, these tumours usually present when they have ulcerated with a raised edge and sometimes a central scab. They are common on the face (Fig. 13), dorsum of the hand, ear and lips. Biopsy confirms the diagnosis and treatment is usually by adequate excision (sometimes with radiotherapy). If neglected these tumours metastasize.

Malignant melanoma

Malignant melanoma (Fig. 14) is relatively rare, but the incidence is increased by prolonged exposure to sunlight. Many arise in pre-existing naevi. Suspect malignancy if a pigmented skin lesion increases in size, changes colour (darker or lighter), bleeds, ulcerates, becomes painful, or develops surrounding satellite lesions. Always examine regional lymph nodes for spread. Treatment is by excision and skin grafting. Prognosis depends on microscopic depth of invasion and on extent of spread, although distant metastases can occur years after treatment.

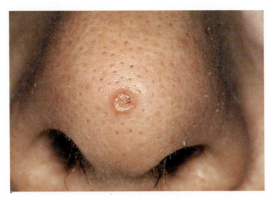

Fig. 12 Basal cell carcinoma on nose.

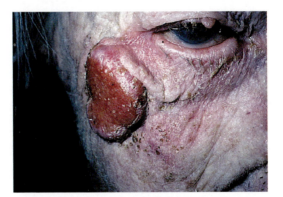

Fig. 13 Squamous cell carcinoma near eye.

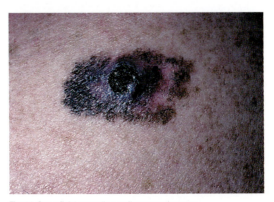

Fig. 14 Superficial spreading malignant melanoma.

2 / Nails

Ingrowing toenail This is a very common condition that most often affects the hallux (Fig. 15). The distal edge of the nail grows into the nail fold, producing chronic infection with redness, swelling, pain, and intermittent discharge of pus. Acute paronychia requires drainage by removal of the nail. Persistent trouble may demand radical excision of the nail bed as well. In either case excision of a wedge of nail or bed on the affected side will suffice.

Onychogryphosis Onychogryphosis is commoner with increasing age. One or more nails (most often the hallux, Fig. 16) become grossly thickened, deformed, and hypertrophic. Chiropody may suffice as treatment, but nail bed excision is required for cure.

Health lines (Beau's lines) These transverse depressions affect all the nails symmetrically (Fig. 17) and result from an episode of severe general illness which disturbs nail growth. The lines move distally as the nails grow.

Clubbing There are many causes of clubbing, including congenital cyanotic heart disease, bronchial carcinoma, chronic chest sepsis, cirrhosis and inflammatory bowel disease. Initially the angle between the proximal nail fold and the nail is lost. The tissues beneath the nail and the finger pulp then become obviously swollen and finally the end of the finger swells laterally to produce a 'drumstick' appearance (Fig. 18).

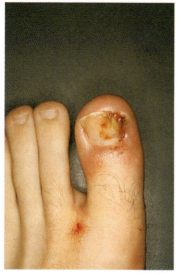

Fig. 15 Ingrowing toenail of hallux.

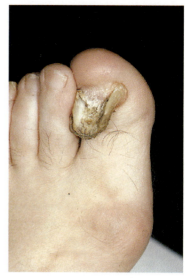

Fig. 16 Onychogryphosis of hallux.

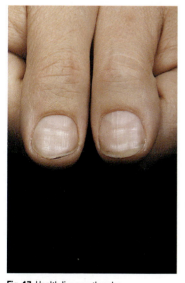

Fig. 17 Health lines on thumbs.

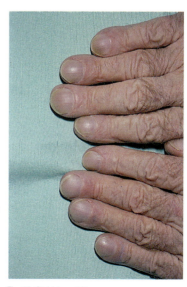

Fig. 18 Clubbing of fingers.

3 / Cervical lymph nodes

Full examination of the cervical lymph nodes requires inspection and palpation both from in front and behind. It is useful to palpate from the point of the chin back to the angle of the jaw. Continue down the line of the jugular vein and then include both anterior and posterior triangles. Nodes also lie both anterior and posterior to the ear. Enlargement of any of the nodes should lead to a search for a primary source of malignancy or infection. Any area of the head or neck may be the site; supraclavicular nodes can enlarge secondary to tumours of the stomach or bronchus. Specific examples include:

Hodgkin's disease

This form of lymphoma commonly presents with a single focus in the neck (Fig. 19). The enlarged nodes are discrete and non-tender. A search should be made in axillae and groins as well as an abdominal examination for hepatomegaly or splenomegaly. Fine needle aspiration cytology suggests the diagnosis, but open biopsy will be required to establish it.

Cervical abscess

Cervical abscesses are uncommon due to early use of antibiotics.

If untreated, infected lymph nodes will eventually liquefy to form an abscess. In the neck this is initially confined by the deep cervical fascia. Eventually it will break through, forming a collar-stud abscess (Fig. 20). This will require drainage. Healing may be prolonged as the track may be long and tortuous.

Tuberculous adenitis

Nowadays this condition is uncommon in the West, though it is still prevalent in some parts of the world. Differential diagnosis from malignancy is often difficult initially. The tonsillar node is usually the first to be involved. Diagnosis is by biopsy and culture. Untreated inflammation of a node will eventually lead to an abscess (Fig. 21).

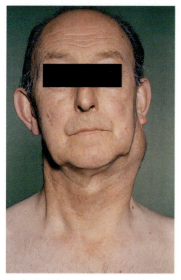

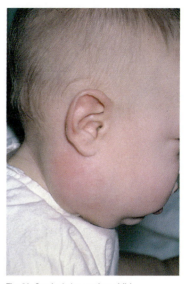

Fig. 19 Hodgkin's disease in cervical lymph nodes.

Fig. 20 Cervical abscess in a child.

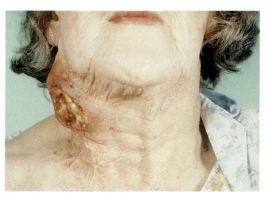

Fig. 21 Tuberculous lymphadenitis of neck.

4 / Secondary malignancy

Metastases in lymph nodes
The neck is a common site for secondary malignancy. This should always be considered if hard nodes are palpated, and a generalized examination performed. A chest X-ray is essential. Fine needle aspiration cytology is a major asset.

The finding of squamous carcinoma suggests mouth and pharynx as the primary site, whilst adenocarcinoma may arise from lung or stomach. However, not all secondary malignancy is found in lymph nodes.

Skin nodules
These metastatic nodules, which vary from single to widespread, are numerous and may be the first sign of malignancy (Fig. 22). They seem to appear rapidly and vary greatly in size. Excision biopsy under a local anaesthetic is a simple diagnostic technique.

Typical tumours to produce these findings include breast and bronchus.

Bony metastases
Secondary malignancy in bone (Fig. 23) will usually present with pain or a pathological fracture. Occasionally, however, it will present as a mass lesion. If clinical examination and radiology (Fig. 24) do not identify the source then a core biopsy should make histological diagnosis feasible.

Tumours that commonly metastasize to bone are breast, bronchus, prostate, thyroid and kidney.

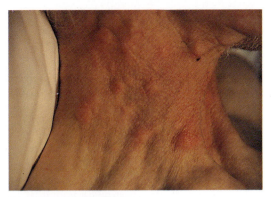

Fig. 22 Metastatic nodules in the skin.

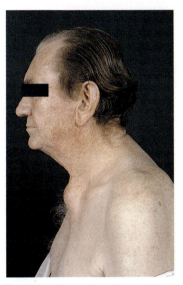

Fig. 23 Secondary carcinoma in manubrium.

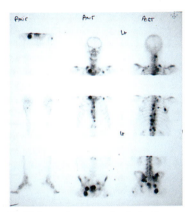

Fig. 24 Isotope bone scan of patient with metastases from carcinoma of the breast.

5 / **Parotid gland**

Parotitis Inflammation of the parotid gland results in a generalized painful enlargement of the whole gland (Fig. 25). There may occasionally be a discharge of pus from the duct orifice which lies above the second upper molar tooth. The infection may be bacterial or viral (e.g. mumps) and can be unilateral or bilateral. Chronic parotitis secondary to calculus disease is usually painless.

Tumours Although any part of the gland can be involved the majority of tumours arise just in front of and above the angle of the jaw. The tragus is lifted up and displaced. The tumour is commonly mistaken for an enlarged preauricular node. Fine needle cytology may help with the diagnosis. Examination must include an assessment of the facial nerve which may be involved.

The following types of tumour occur:

Mixed parotid tumour (pleomorphic adenoma): the commonest type (Fig. 26). Often growing to a large size they tend to recur locally, but rarely undergo frank malignant change. They should be resected, usually with the entire superficial portion of the gland before malignancy intervenes; the facial nerve should be identified and preserved (Fig. 27).

Adenolymphomas: less common and often softer to the touch (Fig. 28). Diagnosis is essentially histological.

Carcinomas: account for 10% of parotid tumours and may be primary or secondary to a pleomorphic adenoma. The nerve may be involved, producing facial paralysis. Treatment is by resection or radiotherapy. A resected nerve can sometimes be successfully grafted.

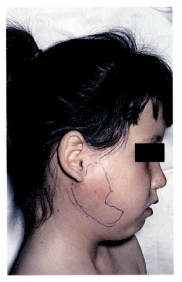

Fig. 25 Acute parotitis in a child.

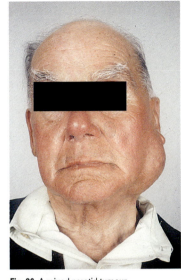

Fig. 26 A mixed parotid tumour.

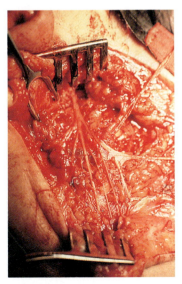

Fig. 27 Facial nerve displayed during superficial parotidectomy.

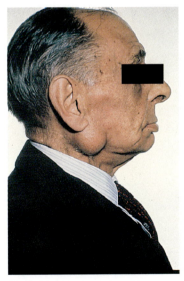

Fig. 28 Adenolymphoma of parotid.

6 / Submandibular gland

The gland has a superficial part and a deep part wrapped around the mylohyoid, and the duct opens under the front of the tongue. When enlarged the gland presents as a swelling below and in front of the angle of the jaw. Bimanual palpation with a finger in the mouth is a useful method of examination.

Tumours Tumours of the submandibular gland are uncommon compared with those of the parotid gland or with chronic sialectasis. The pleomorphic adenoma is the most frequent, presenting as a permanent slowly growing hard swelling (Fig. 29). Radiology should be undertaken to exclude a calculus and treatment is by excision.

Sialectasis Sialectasis is seen most commonly in this gland. The swelling is often intermittent and painful soon after starting to eat. The patient may need to suck a bitter sweet to demonstrate the swelling.

The cause is often a single calculus at the duct orifice in the mouth (Fig. 31). Often palpable or visible they also show on X-ray (Fig. 30). In these cases the stone can be removed under local anaesthetic with consequent relief. More widespread stone disease with destruction of glandular tissue leads to a permanent swelling which requires to be excised. Damage to the lingual nerve must be avoided.

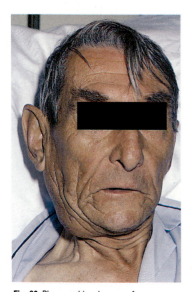

Fig. 29 Pleomorphic adenoma of submandibular gland.

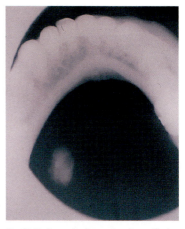

Fig. 30 Radiograph of stone in submandibular duct.

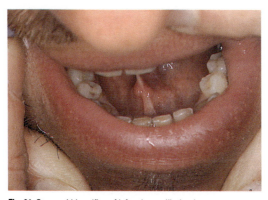

Fig. 31 Stone within orifice of left submandibular duct.

7 / Mouth

Ectopic salivary tumour This is a misnomer as minor salivary glands are scattered over the pharynx and palate and are not truly ectopic. Tumours in these glands are not uncommon and the usual site is the palate (Fig. 32). Initially symptomless, they may ulcerate and become painful. Many are pleomorphic adenomas, but the commonest is the cylindroma. This is a low grade malignant tumour which may invade locally or metastasize.

Ranula A ranula presents as a blue domed swelling in the floor of the mouth (Fig. 33) where it can best be palpated bimanually as it can extend into the neck. It is in fact a cyst of the sublingual gland and is treated by surgical excision.

Telangiectasia Not confined to the face alone, these may be a non-specific marker of systemic disease such as scleroderma (Fig. 34). They may also occur in association with gut telangiectases in the Rendu-Osler-Weber syndrome.

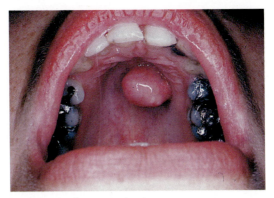

Fig. 32 Ectopic salivary tumour in palate.

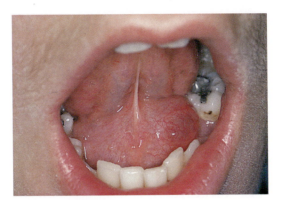

Fig. 33 Ranula in floor of mouth.

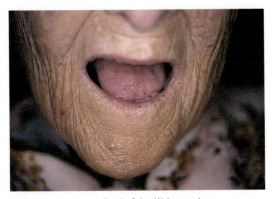

Fig. 34 Telangiectases in Rendu–Osler–Weber syndrome.

Oral candidiasis Oral candidiasis presents as characteristic white plaques with painful ulceration which can cover the tongue and pharynx (Fig. 35). In severe cases the oesophagus becomes involved with consequent dysphagia. It is common in childhood but presents in later life in association with antibiotic usage or malignancy. It is also seen in immunodeficiency states and is increasingly the first feature of HIV infection.

Leukoplakia The normal surface of the tongue is lost and areas of thickened white epithelium appear (Fig. 36). Initially small, the areas have a tendency to enlarge and coalesce. Careful observation and palpation is required as this chronic superficial glossitis may progress to carcinoma. Although not all cases do progress, about one-third of carcinomas arise from leukoplakia.

Carcinoma Carcinoma of the mouth is uncommon. The commonest tumour of the mouth presents on the tongue (Fig. 37). This starts with an ulcer which may be painful. It is usually sited on the side or base of the tongue and is often secondary to chronic inflammation. Diagnosis is by biopsy, and treatment involves surgery and/or radiotherapy.

Other rare ulcerating lesions of the tongue include chancre, gumma and tuberculosis.

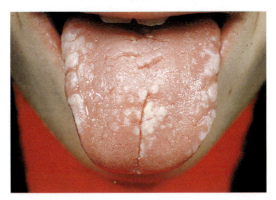

Fig. 35 Oral candidiasis.

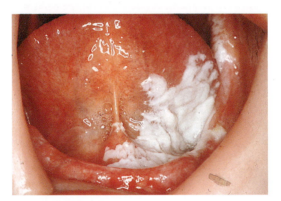

Fig. 36 Leukoplakia of tongue.

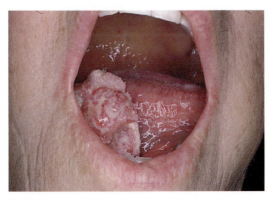

Fig. 37 Squamous carcinoma of tongue.

Deviation of the tongue

When the patient is asked to stick out his tongue lateral deviation may be due to infiltration with carcinoma or hypoglossal nerve palsy.

Infiltration

Unilateral infiltration with carcinoma is the commoner cause of deviation of the tongue. It results in hardness and thickening, which is predominant in one side of the tongue.

Hypoglossal nerve palsy

Hypoglossal nerve lesions cause hemiatrophy of the tongue which deviates towards the paralysed side (Fig. 38). This may be caused by brain stem lesions but can also be a complication of surgery to the neck. The hypoglossal nerve is at risk of damage during operations on the submandibular gland, radical neck dissections for malignancy, and carotid endarterectomy.

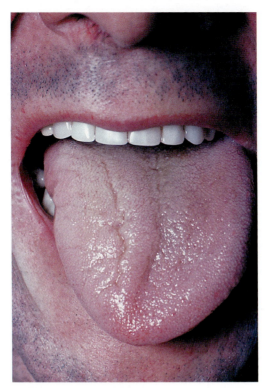

Fig. 38 Hypoglossal nerve palsy.

8 / Branchial lesions

Branchial cyst

Branchial cysts are uncommon. The cyst is thought to be a remnant of the second branchial cleft. Although congenital, presentation is usually delayed until early adult life.

Clinical features Presentation is with a cystic swelling around the anterior border of the sternomastoid, arising deep behind the upper third (Fig. 39). Occasionally they can become infected and present with an abscess that can mimic tuberculosis. Aspiration reveals thin, creamy material with cholesterol crystals on microscopy.

Treatment Treatment is by excision.

Branchial fistula

Branchial fistulae are even less common than branchial cysts and may be bilateral (Fig. 40).

Clinical features A branchial fistula presents as an orifice which lies low and just anterior to the sternomastoid and which discharges soon after birth. The volume of the discharge varies; it is usually thick and sticky. The fistula may occlude, leading to inflammation and infection.

The track itself is usually incomplete reaching only to the pharyngeal wall. Occasionally an internal opening is found behind the tonsil.

Treatment Treatment is by excision. This may necessitate two incisions because of the length and anatomical relationships of the track.

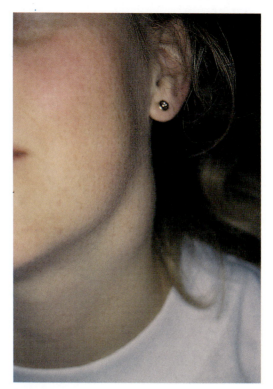

Fig. 39 Branchial cyst.

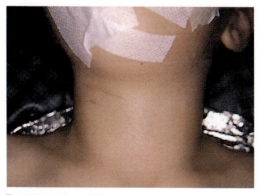

Fig. 40 Bilateral branchial fistulae.

9 / **Thyroid gland**

Thyroglossal cyst

The thyroid gland develops and descends from the area of the foramen caecum at the back of the tongue. It is within this track that a thyroglossal cyst occurs. It can appear at any time of life, but is often first seen in childhood.

Clinical features   A midline swelling is visible which can be separated from the thyroid gland itself (Figs 41 & 42). The key diagnostic feature is the attachment to the base of the tongue. The patient is observed and the swelling is palpated with the mouth open. When the tongue is protruded the cyst moves upwards. Usually close to the thyroid gland, the cyst can occur anywhere along the track.

Treatment   Thyroglossal cysts are liable to infection (Fig. 43) and should therefore be excised, together with the track. This may involve resection of the mid part of the hyoid bone around which the track loops.

Thyroglossal fistula

Aetiology   This midline orifice (Fig. 44) can result from spontaneous discharge of an infected thyroglossal cyst. More commonly it follows excision or drainage of a cyst without removal of the track.

Clinical features   The orifice weeps intermittently and often becomes inflamed.

Treatment   Cure is achieved by excising the entire track.

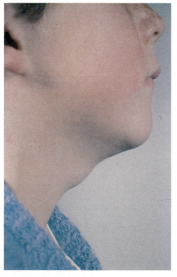

Fig. 41 Lateral view of thyroglossal cyst.

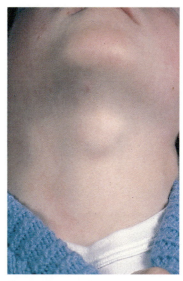

Fig. 42 Anterior view of thyroglossal cyst.

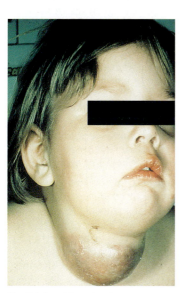

Fig. 43 Infected thyroglossal cyst.

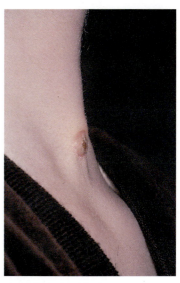

Fig. 44 Thyroglossal fistula.

Goitre

A thyroid swelling (goitre; Fig. 45) should be inspected from in front and palpated from behind. It moves upwards with the larynx on swallowing and then descends. A goitre is best felt with the neck slightly flexed. Initial examination should be to determine whether there is a focal swelling in the gland or whether there is a diffuse swelling of the entire thyroid. Occasionally a large goitre will descend behind the manubrium; this is detected by palpation in the suprasternal notch and percussion over the manubrium. Clinical examination can be complemented by ultrasound and occasionally radio-isotope scanning.

Unilateral goitre

Adenoma: The commonest lesion, which is harmless and can be left if asymptomatic. However, it is frequently impossible to differentiate these lesions clinically from thyroid malignancy. A rapid change in size or hardness of the gland must raise this possibility; in advanced cases the gland may become fixed, with tracheal compression and voice change.

Thyroid carcinoma: frequently presents at a young age, when it is usually papillary in type and often curable. Follicular tumours are intermediate with advanced (anaplastic) tumours occurring in later life. Treatment includes surgery and thyroxine therapy to suppress TSH.

Haemorrhage into a nodular goitre: occasionally presents with the sudden appearance of a large single nodule which can be diagnosed and relieved by aspiration.

Diffuse goitre

Diffuse thyroid enlargement: common around puberty. It should regress within a year or two.

Multinodular goitre: classically endemic in areas where the water is deficient in iodine. The goitre enlarges and becomes obviously multinodular (Fig. 46). Hard change in a nodule raises the possibility of calcification or malignancy, both of which can occur in long-standing disease.

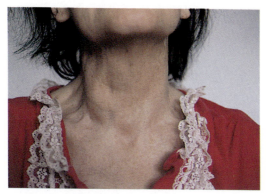

Fig. 45 Goitre affecting right lobe of thyroid.

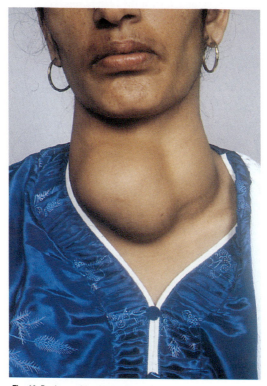

Fig. 46 Benign multinodular goitre.

Thyrotoxicosis

This may be primary with diffuse enlargement of the gland (Graves' disease) or arise secondarily in an adenoma or multinodular goitre. Patients are usually young females.

Clinical features The skin feels warm and the palms are sweaty. The pulse rate is increased and atrial fibrillation is common in older patients; sleeping pulse rate can differentiate from anxiety-induced tachycardia. There is a loss of weight despite good appetite and a fine tremor when the hands are extended with the fingers splayed. Normal reflexes are exaggerated and irritability is often reported.

Eye changes: result from varying degrees of exophthalmos and ophthalmoplegia. Protrusion of the eye results from intra-orbital fat deposition and is accentuated by lid retraction (Fig. 47). The eyes bulge when viewed from above. When asked to follow a finger slowly up and down, the upper lid lags. The staring gaze increases as the exophthalmos progresses; occasionally this may occur even after successful treatment of thyrotoxicosis. Pretibial myxoedema may rarely occur on the shin in thyrotoxicosis (Fig. 48).

Myxoedema

Clinical features The symptoms and signs of myxoedema are the reverse of thyrotoxicosis. The hands are cold, the eyelids and the face puffy. The hair thins, the skin is waxy and there may be a malar flush. The pulse is slow, as are the thought processes. The neck should be examined for fatty deposits in the supraclavicular fossa. The tissues in general may feel firm with the development of pseudo-oedema. Although these are the classical changes of myxoedema the majority of patients have no obvious features and myxoedema is largely a serum diagnosis.

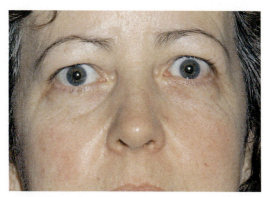

Fig. 47 Thyrotoxic facies.

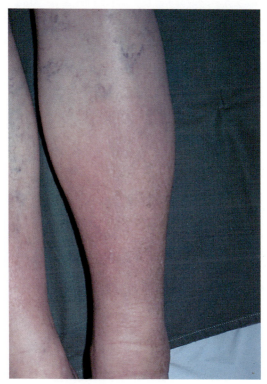

Fig. 48 Pretibial myxoedema.

10 / Breast

Examination Examination of the breast should commence with the patient naked to the waist and sitting upright. Attention should be paid to the shape, contours, texture of the skin and nipples. Raising the arms may reveal nipple retraction or skin dimpling by an adherent malignancy. Palpation with the flats of the fingers is performed with the patient supine and should include the axillae and supraclavicular fossae; start with the normal breast.

Benign lump

Clinical types **Fibroadenoma**: the commonest solitary lump, and most frequent in younger women. The lump is smooth and rounded and moves easily under the fingers—it is sometimes called a breast 'mouse'. Clinical diagnosis alone is unwise and should be supported by benign aspiration cytology if the lump is not to be excised.

Fibroadenosis: a more diffuse change and the most common cause of a lump in the breast. Often generalized, it may be confined to one quadrant of the breast. The lump or lumpiness is usually tender and changes in size and shape with the menstrual cycle; being least 5–7 days after the start of a period. If the clinical diagnosis is uncertain then re-examination at a different stage of the cycle may be useful. If in doubt, however, biopsy should be advised. Mammography may be useful, but is of limited value in young women (Fig. 49).

Breast cyst

Breast cysts are common, usually arising in a setting of fibroadenosis.

Clinical features The cyst is usually very firm but rounded and smooth. Careful examination may reveal a suspicion of fluctuation but this can be misleading.

Investigations All solitary lumps should be aspirated (Fig. 50) and no further treatment is required if the fluid is not bloodstained, the lump disappears, and the cyst does not refill on re-examination. The colour of the fluid varies but, unless bloody, cytology is of no value.

Treatment Cysts should be excised if they recur twice.

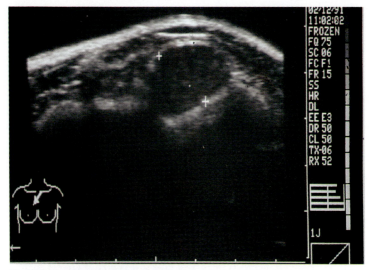

Fig. 49 Benign breast lump: ultrasound scan.

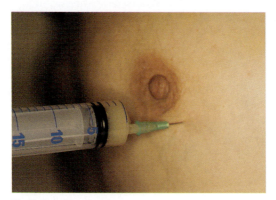

Fig. 50 Aspiration of breast cyst.

Conditions affecting the nipple

Nipple discharge

A question about nipple discharge should be routine. If present the colour, frequency and site of the discharge should be noted. Fibroadenosis (Fig. 51) and duct ectasia produce a discharge which may be clear, green, or yellow. Bleeding is almost always from a single duct and most frequently due to a benign duct papilloma. Careful examination of the breast is required to exclude a carcinoma. All nipple discharges should be sent for cytology which will frequently help with a diagnosis. The appearance of the discharge from both breasts or multiple ducts suggests benign disease.

Nipple retraction

Initially this may occur at puberty when the nipple is tethered as the breast grows. It is vital therefore to ask the patient if retraction is recent. Retraction in later life (Fig. 52) is most often due to fibroadenosis, but can be a sign of malignancy. If associated with a lump biopsy is usually required.

Paget's disease

Classically Paget's disease of the nipple presents as an eczematous rash (Fig. 53). However, dry scaly skin around the nipple, with itching also suggests the possibility of Paget's disease. The changes result from malignant invasion of the lymphatics under the nipple.

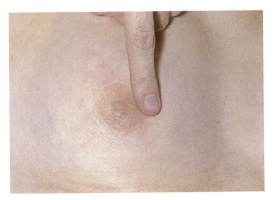

Fig. 51 Nipple discharge in fibroadenosis.

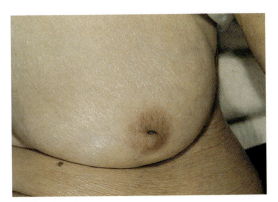

Fig. 52 Retracted nipple.

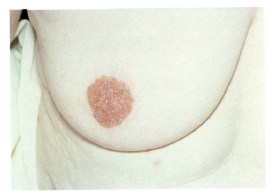

Fig. 53 Paget's disease of the nipple.

Mastitis

Mastitis, or inflammation of the breast, may occur in infants soon after birth and also at puberty. In both instances it can affect boys as well as girls and is usually self-limiting. Although probably hormonal it is curiously usually unilateral.

Acute bacterial mastitis can occur secondary to fibroadenosis, but is most commonly seen in lactating women.

Clinical features An area of the breast becomes swollen, hot and tender. The organism is most commonly *Staphylococcus aureus* and abscess formation is common (Fig. 54).

Treatment Once pus has formed surgical drainage is required. Antibiotics may occasionally sterilize an abscess leading to an 'antibioma' which may be difficult to distinguish from a carcinoma; ultrasound scanning is often diagnostic.

If the history is rather prolonged, or the breast not as tender as expected, the possibility of an inflammatory carcinoma must be considered.

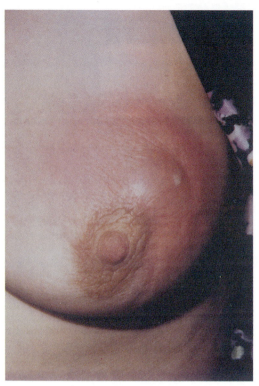

Fig. 54 Breast abscess.

Accessory tissue   The nipple line runs from the axilla down the anterior chest and abdomen and into the groin. The presence of one or more vestigial nipples (Fig. 55) along this line is not uncommon and they are often mistaken for skin papillomata. The development of an accessory breast (Fig. 56) is unusual, but they may even lactate if fully formed.

Gynaecomastia   **At puberty**. Enlargement of the breast tissue in a male (Fig. 57) is often seen at puberty and may be bilateral or unilateral. The condition is usually self-limiting with regression after 6–12 months. Surgery may be required if it persists and the tissue is tender or socially embarrassing.

In later life. Enlargement of the breast tissue can occur secondary to testicular tumours, or with the development of fibroadenosis. A careful drug history may be taken as gynaecomastia is often drug induced. Benign disease presents as a round, smooth disc directly behind the nipple, which should distinguish it from carcinoma, which is often slightly eccentric.

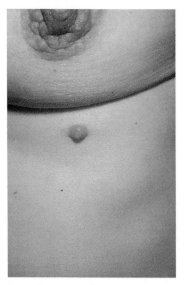

Fig. 55 Accessory nipple.

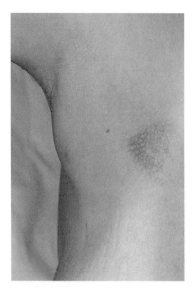

Fig. 56 Accessory breast in axilla.

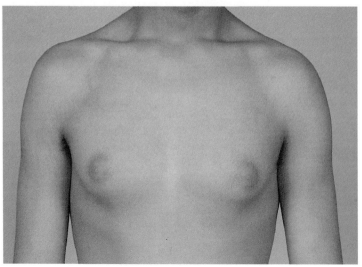

Fig. 57 Gynaecomastia in a young man.

Carcinoma

Most women presenting with a lump in the breast are concerned that they have a carcinoma. The general principles of examination have been described earlier (see p. 33).

Clinical features

Breast cancers present with a lump that is typically hard and irregular. The commonest sites are the upper outer quadrants and behind the nipple. Fixity to the skin (Figs 58 & 59) should be assessed by palpation. Deep tethering can be diagnosed by asking the patient to contract the pectoral muscles by pressing the hands against the hips. Skin oedema secondary to lymphatic permeation produces the characteristic sign of peau d'orange (Fig. 62, p. 44). Advanced cases will eventually ulcerate through the skin.

Investigations

All breast lumps merit needle aspiration for cytology. The feel of the needle entering the lump may well assist the clinical diagnosis. Cytology is diagnostic if positive and permits the clinician to discuss the treatment options prior to surgery.

Examination of lymph nodes

Treatment and prognosis depend on the staging of the tumour. Although this may be altered by the histological results it can be undertaken using the TNM classification (see p. 43). Examination of the axillae and supraclavicular fossae is mandatory. The axillae are examined by lifting the patient's arm and passing the fingertips high into the apex of the axilla. The arm is returned to the patient's side and the examining hand can then palpate the contents of the axilla against the lateral chest wall. For this manoeuvre it is essential that the examiner takes the weight of the patient's arm to relax the surrounding muscles. Finally, the pectoral and supraclavicular areas should be examined.

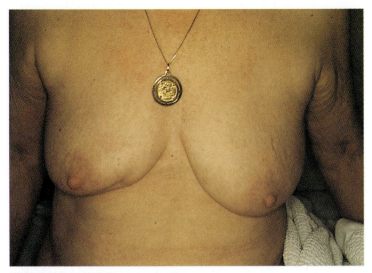

Fig. 58 Carcinoma of right breast, arms by sides.

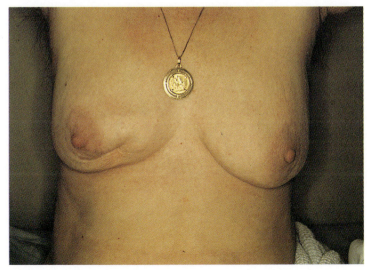

Fig. 59 Same patient as in Figure 58 with arms elevated: note increased skin retraction.

Staging of breast carcinoma

As with all malignancy, breast carcinoma is routinely staged to reflect the size, nodal status and metastatic character of the presenting disease. This helps not only in planning therapy but also in determining the prognosis of the patient at hand. It is also vital when comparing patients in clinical trials. Below is the TNM classification for carcinoma of the breast.

Size
T_1—2 cm diameter or less, no skin fixation
T_2—more than 2 cm but less than 5 cm; or—less than 2 cm with skin tethering
T_3—more than 5 cm but less than 10 cm; or—less than 5 cm with skin tethering
T_4—any size of tumour with infiltration or ulceration of the skin wide of the tumour (Figs 60 & 61); or—peau d'orange (Fig. 62); or—chest wall fixation

Nodal status
N_0—no palpable axillary nodes
N_1—palpable mobile axillary nodes
N_2—fixed axillary nodes
N_3—palpable supraclavicular nodes

Metastatic character
M_0—no evidence of distant metastases
M_1—distant metastases anywhere

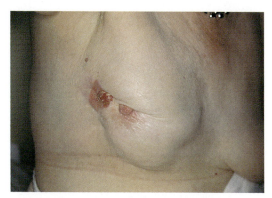

Fig. 60 Fungating carcinoma of breast.

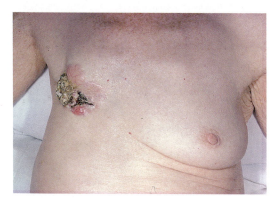

Fig. 61 Fungating carcinoma with destruction of breast.

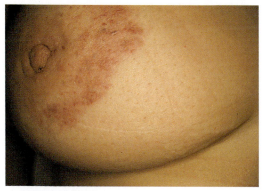

Fig. 62 Peau d'orange.

11 / Intestinal obstruction

Aetiology The commonest causes of small bowel obstruction are postoperative adhesions (look for scars) or hernias (never miss a small femoral hernia in an obstructed, elderly woman). In the large bowel, carcinoma is the commonest cause.

Clinical features The four cardinal features are:
- colicky pain
- vomiting
- abdominal distension
- constipation.

Small bowel obstruction: vomiting occurs early, distension is rarely gross and tends to be central and constipation is uncommon. Visible peristalsis is sometimes a feature (Fig. 64).

Large bowel obstruction: huge distension may occur, perhaps more marked initially in the flanks (Fig. 63), vomiting is later and less common, while constipation occurs early and may be absolute (no faeces or flatus).

Features suggesting strangulation of the bowel are constant, unremitting pain, tachycardia, and peritonism. These demand early operation.

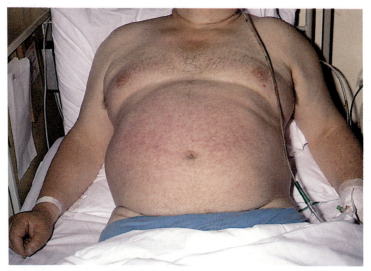
Fig. 63 Distended abdomen in intestinal obstruction.

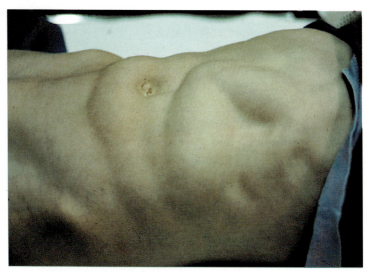
Fig. 64 Visible peristalsis in small bowel obstruction.

Plain X-rays   Plain abdominal radiographs aid the diagnosis of
intestinal obstruction and help to determine the site.

Small bowel: tends to lie centrally, sometimes produces
a 'ladder pattern' of adjacent distended loops, and has
transverse shadows crossing its whole width produced by
the circular mucosal folds (Figs 65 & 66).

Large bowel: tends to lie peripherally and shows the
indentations of the haustral folds, but no complete
transverse bands (Fig. 67).

Traditionally, supine and erect views are taken, the
latter showing classic 'fluid levels' (Fig. 66) of obstructed
small bowel (also seen in paralytic ileus or
gastroenteritis). Distended bowel is seen in either view.
The distal extent of distended bowel suggests the site of
obstruction. Gross distension of the caecum can occur
with a competent ileocaecal valve and suggests the risk of
caecal rupture.

Sigmoid volvulus

In sigmoid volvulus a long and mobile loop of sigmoid
colon twists on its mesentery producing rapid gross
distension. The radiograph shows an inverted 'omega
loop' often with two fluid levels (Fig. 68). Sigmoid
volvulus occurs more frequently in elderly, constipated
men. It is common in parts of Africa and Asia.

Treatment   Early treatment is vital—either decompression with a
rectal tube or colonoscope, or else by laparotomy.

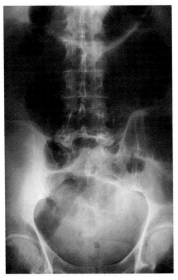

Fig. 65 Small bowel obstruction: supine X-ray.

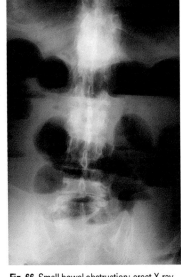

Fig. 66 Small bowel obstruction: erect X-ray.

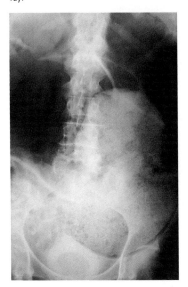

Fig. 67 Large bowel obstruction.

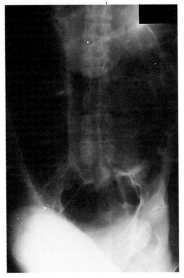

Fig. 68 Radiograph of sigmoid volvulus.

12 / Ascites

Aetiology   Common causes of ascites in surgical practice are disseminated intra-abdominal malignancy (especially from ovary and bowel) and liver disease. Cirrhosis is the commonest hepatic cause and produces ascites by the effects of portal hypertension, hypo-albuminaemia, and salt and water retention. Any general cause of extravascular fluid accumulation may also cause ascites (e.g. chronic heart failure, renal failure, severe malnutrition).

Clinical features   Ascites causes generalized abdominal distension (Figs 69 & 70). Percussion over the uppermost part of the abdominal wall will be resonant due to bowel. If the patient then turns on to his side percussion over the same area becomes dull, as fluid gravitates to this part of the peritoneal cavity (Fig. 70). This sign is called 'shifting dullness'.

A classic sign of ascites is a fluid thrill. The examiner flicks one side of the abdominal wall and feels the thrill transmitted through ascitic fluid to the opposite side. An assistant with his hand placed firmly in the midline prevents transmission of a thrill through the fat of the abdominal wall.

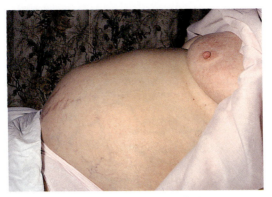

Fig. 69 Abdomen distended by ascites (lateral view).

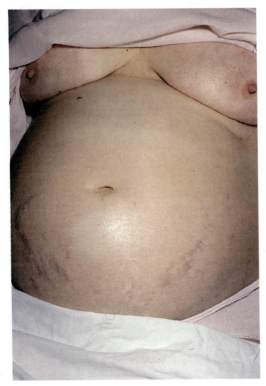

Fig. 70 Same patient as in Figure 69 (anterior view): note abdominal striae.

13 / **Jaundice**

Jaundice results from the build-up of bilirubin within the body, which may be prehepatic (e.g. haemolytic anaemias), hepatic (e.g. hepatitis) or post-hepatic (obstructive).

Obstructive jaundice

Clinical features   Presentation occurs first with a yellow tinge to the sclerae of the eyes (Fig. 71). It is rarely visible unless the bilirubin is at least twice the upper limit of normal. As jaundice deepens, the skin becomes yellow (Fig. 72) and the onset of itching leads to excoriation. The urine becomes dark and the stools pale (Fig. 73). The two commonest causes are gallstones and malignancy.

Gallstones. These are common and usually associated with a recent attack of biliary colic. The level of jaundice may fluctuate from day to day. Jaundice is usually due to a stone in the common bile duct but can also result from cholangitis. In cholangitis the patient is pyrexial and may have rigors. The gallbladder is usually impalpable but the right upper quadrant is tender.

Malignancy. Obstructive jaundice caused by malignancy is most commonly due to pancreatic carcinoma. The jaundice is usually progressive and does not fluctuate. Although clinically painless, most patients have a degree of epigastric discomfort that radiates to the back and can be severe. Examination of the abdomen may reveal a smooth, enlarged and non-tender gallbladder. Courvoisier's law states that if the gallbladder is enlarged in a jaundiced patient then the jaundice is unlikely to be due to stone. Exceptions include a gallbladder with stones which is fibrosed and incapable of distension. In advanced cases a pancreatic tumour may be palpable. All jaundiced patients lose weight, but this is most pronounced with malignancy.

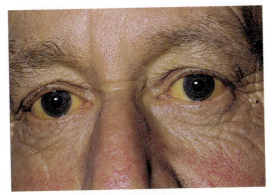

Fig. 71 Icteric sclerae in obstructive jaundice.

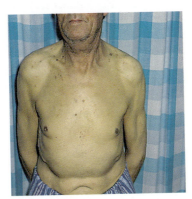

Fig. 72 A jaundiced patient.

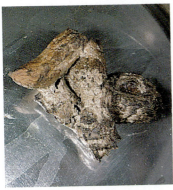
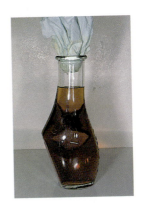

Fig. 73 Faeces and urine in obstructive jaundice.

Obstructive jaundice (contd)

Investigations   Serum tests give a rapid and reliable estimation of the severity of the jaundice and provide a likely pointer as to whether or not it is obstructive. Viral titres can be assessed and clotting function, often deranged, should be monitored.

Radiology. An ultrasound scan is an essential early step in assessment of the jaundiced patient. It demonstrates whether or not the bile ducts are dilated (Fig. 74), and may well show the cause of obstruction. If gallstones are demonstrated (Fig. 75) they may, or may not, be the cause of jaundice. CT scanning provides more accurate information. Tumours as small as 5 mm are usually visible. Contrast enhancement may reveal involvement of the major vessels and predict resectability.

Endoscopic retrograde cholangiopancreatography (ERCP). ERCP is increasingly important for the diagnosis of jaundice and may be followed by a therapeutic procedure such as sphincterotomy. It has largely replaced percutaneous transhepatic cholangiography (Fig. 76) for diagnosis and also for sphincterotomy and stenting.

Treatment   Sphincterotomy enables stones to be extracted and the jaundice relieved. Cholecystectomy may then be performed laparoscopically. In malignant obstructive jaundice a stent can be inserted, either to provide good palliation, or more rarely to restore normal hepatic function and improve the prospects for surgical resection of the tumour.

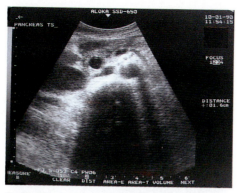

Fig. 74 Dilated common bile duct (top left with markers).

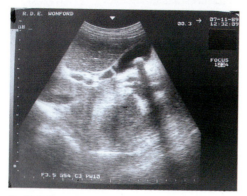

Fig. 75 Gallstones in gallbladder.

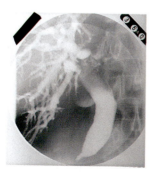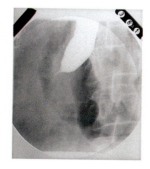

Fig. 76 Percutaneous transhepatic cholangiogram showing an obstructed common bile duct.

14 / Vena caval obstruction

Superior vena cava

Obstruction of the superior vena cava is usually the result of a tumour in the posterior mediastinum.

Clinical features The veins in the head and neck become swollen and engorged. The skin may take on a cyanotic hue and oedema of the face is also a feature.

Inferior vena cava

Pressure from an intra-abdominal mass or direct invasion by adenocarcinoma of the kidney can obstruct the inferior vena cava.

Clinical features The veins of the lower abdominal wall become full (Fig. 77). The key to the diagnosis is the direction of flow. Normally veins on the lower abdominal wall drain inferiorly, whereas in inferior vena caval obstruction flow is reversed. Using two fingers a segment of vein can be flattened and emptied, and the direction of flow can be observed as it refills. Distension with downward flow may rarely be due to portal hypertension.

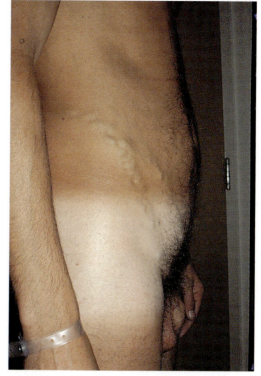

Fig. 77 Dilated abdominal wall veins in inferior vena caval obstruction.

15 / **Abdominal trauma**

Injuries to the abdomen may result from penetrating or blunt trauma.

Penetrating abdominal trauma
Injuries resulting from stabbings or gunshot wounds remain uncommon in the United Kingdom. Whilst the extent of the trauma may be impossible to determine prior to surgery there is no doubt that an injury has occurred.

Blunt abdominal trauma
Blunt abdominal trauma (Fig. 78) is more difficult to define, particularly when associated with a head injury which may render the patient unconscious. The patient or an accompanying person may be able to give a clear picture of how the injury occurred. The signs are both general and local.

General signs General signs are those of hypovolaemia. The patient is pale, in pain, with a tachycardia and often tachypnoea. He feels cold, clammy and peripherally shut-down.

Local signs Local signs are those of peritonism; tenderness and guarding which may be diffuse, or localized to the injured area. Diaphragmatic irritation will produce pain localized to the shoulders. Clothing marks on the skin indicate a high impact injury where the abdominal wall has been crushed against the spine; a laparotomy is required. Blood may also be revealed by discolouration of the umbilicus (Fig. 79). The development of subcapsular haematomas (Fig. 80) means that frank rupture may be delayed for days or weeks after splenic or liver injury.

Investigations The use of peritoneal lavage and ultrasound scanning will help define the diagnosis in the difficult case.

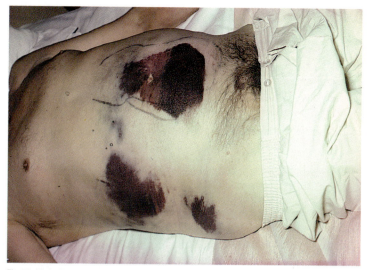

Fig. 78 Marked abdominal wall bruising following a road traffic accident.

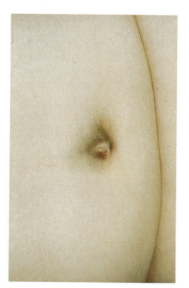

Fig. 79 Cullen's sign: bloodstaining presenting at the umbilicus.

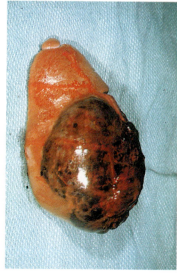

Fig. 80 A subcapsular haematoma of the spleen.

16 / **Pancreas**

Acute pancreatitis

Aetiology   The commonest causes of acute pancreatitis are gall-stones and alcohol.

Clinical features   Acute pancreatitis presents as an acute abdominal emergency with severe epigastric pain radiating to the back. Vomiting is common. Examination reveals abdominal tenderness and guarding, maximal in the upper abdomen. Pulse rate is increased and the blood pressure often low. Mild cyanosis and jaundice are frequently present. The symptoms and signs are similar to those of a perforated peptic ulcer.

Investigations   Diagnosis can usually be made on the basis of a serum amylase investigation.

Prognosis   Whilst most attacks resolve rapidly with supportive therapy some cases progress to a severe and fatal illness.

Prognostication can be performed on the basis of a set of serum tests; the Glasgow criteria. The development of staining in the flanks (Grey Turner's sign; Fig. 81) is of poor prognostic significance. An alternative technique is peritoneal aspiration and lavage; the darker the colour of the fluid aspirated (Fig. 82), the worse the outcome.

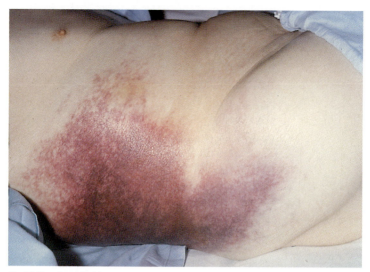

Fig. 81 Grey Turner's sign.

lavage fluid

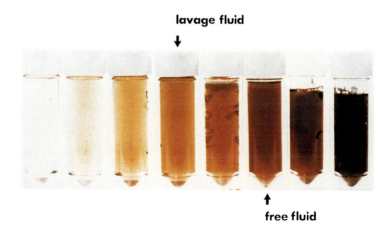

free fluid

Fig. 82 Grading a chart of peritoneal fluid in acute pancreatitis.

Pancreatic cysts

Pancreatic cysts can form in both acute and chronic pancreatitis.

Cysts in acute pancreatitis
These are pseudocysts due to a collection of pancreatic juice outside the pancreas, usually in the lesser sac.

Clinical features Ultrasound scanning (Fig. 84) has revealed these cysts to be common, usually asymptomatic and liable to resolve spontaneously. If they enlarge and become visible (Fig. 83) or palpable they will usually cause pressure symptoms on the stomach (Fig. 85) or duodenum.

Treatment Treatment is initially by ultrasound guided aspiration, but if this fails surgical drainage into stomach or small bowel may be required. Occasionally infection supervenes, the cyst becomes tender and the patient becomes unwell—external drainage is then required.

Cysts in chronic pancreatitis
Clinical features A chronic relapsing and debilitating disease manifest by pain and eventually by both exocrine and endocrine pancreatic failure. Cysts occur as enlargements of the pancreatic duct. They may be large enough to be visible and palpable in an undernourished patient.

Treatment Treatment by drainage into a jejunal loop may relieve some of the pain.

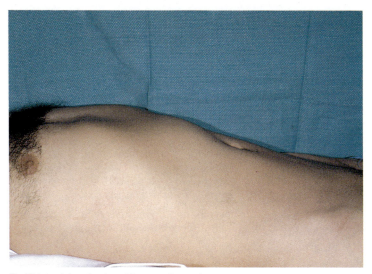

Fig. 83 Lateral view of patient with pancreatic pseudocyst.

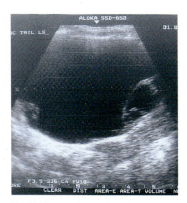

Fig. 84 Ultrasound scan of pancreatic pseudocyst.

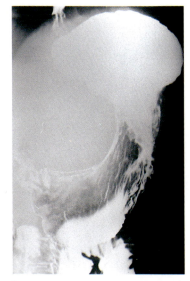

Fig. 85 Barium meal showing compression of stomach.

17 / Ovarian cyst

Ovarian cysts are common. They may be benign or malignant and are usually unilateral.

Clinical features Ovarian cysts are frequently small and only felt by vaginal examination or seen on a pelvic ultrasound scan.

When large, an ovarian cyst rises out of the pelvis to become palpable and often visible (Fig. 86). Its shape and mobility to palpation make the diagnosis fairly easy. It can be distinguished from omental cysts which only move across the line of their mesentery.

Investigations Ultrasound scanning (Fig. 87) is usually diagnostic and often indicates whether the cyst is benign or malignant.

Treatment Treatment is by surgical excision (Fig. 88).

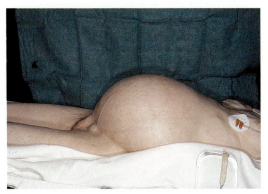

Fig. 86 Abdomen distended by a huge ovarian cyst.

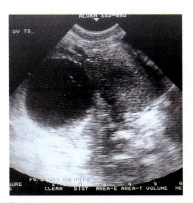

Fig. 87 Ultrasound scan of ovarian cyst.

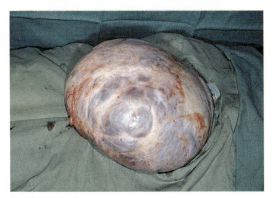

Fig. 88 Large benign ovarian cyst at operation.

18 / Urinary tract

Retention of urine

Retention of urine is most commonly due to benign prostatic hypertrophy and is also frequently seen after major surgery.

Clinical features
The patient presents in distress and unable to pass urine.

The bladder may be visible as a suprapubic swelling, often best seen on inspection from the side (Fig. 89). Palpation reveals a firm mass arising centrally out of the pelvis, which is dull to percussion, and tender. Rectal examination may not be informative until the bladder has been decompressed.

Treatment
Urethral or suprapubic catheterization gives immediate relief.

Renal tumours

Clinical features
Children. Renal malignancy in childhood is uncommon and usually presents with an abdominal swelling. Approximately one-third of cases present with haematuria.

Adults. In adult life adenocarcinoma of the kidney most commonly presents with painless but intermittent haematuria. This warning sign should lead to investigation prior to the development of a mass.

Investigations
Detection is usually by a combination of intravenous pyelography and ultrasound scanning. The tumour has a habit of invading and growing up the renal veins. Should this obstruct the venous return from the gonad in the male then a varicocele may develop (Fig. 90) and act as a further early warning sign. Urine cytology may be of additional value.

Treatment
Treatment is by radical nephrectomy.

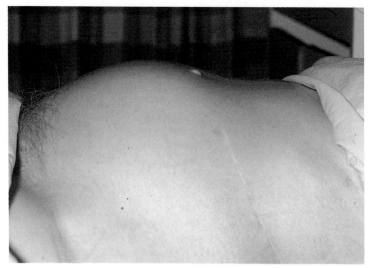

Fig. 89 Painful distended bladder in acute retention of urine.

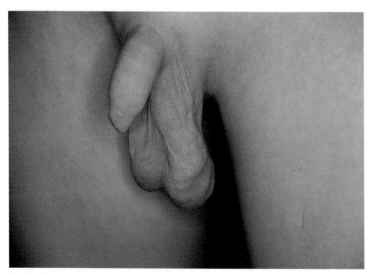

Fig. 90 A left sided varicocele: a potential warning sign of a carcinoma of the kidney.

19 / Appendicitis

Clinical features   **Presentation**: with acute abdominal pain. This starts centrally and slowly becomes more localized. The patient feels generally unwell with anorexia, nausea, vomiting.

Signs: initially few, with only a mild rise in pulse and temperature; abdominal inspection reveals nothing. Palpation should commence as for all acute abdomens away from the site of the pain. Localized tenderness and rigidity are maximal over McBurney's point. Pressure over the left iliac fossa may produce pain on the right side (Rovsing's sign). If the appendix lies behind the ileum or caecum the signs may be less florid. Rectal examination is an essential part of the assessment of a patient with suspected appendicitis—tenderness is especially marked if the appendix lies in the pelvis. If perforation occurs the signs intensify, peritonitis becomes generalized, and the patient becomes profoundly unwell.

Appendix mass
Occasionally a patient presents late in the illness, when omentum and bowel have become adherent around the inflamed appendix.

Clinical features   On abdominal examination a mass is found in the right iliac fossa. Its size may be measured and its extent marked on the abdominal wall.

Treatment   If the patient is not toxic antibiotics can be given and if the mass resolves (Fig. 91) surgery can be delayed or avoided altogether.

Psoas abscess
If an inflamed appendix lies on psoas major, then psoas spasm causes flexion of the hip joint (Fig. 92).

Clinical features   Attempted extension of the hip causes pain and the patient may be unable to walk. An abscess may develop within the psoas sheath itself and track down to present in the groin.

Although psoas abscess may present in appendicitis it was classically due to tuberculosis of the spine. The commonest cause in the Western world at present is probably Crohn's disease.

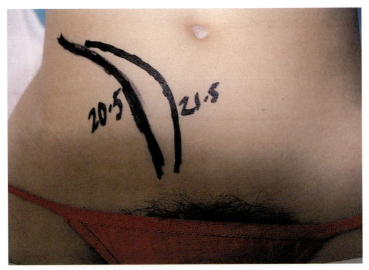

Fig. 91 Measurement lines showing resolution of appendix mass with conservative therapy.

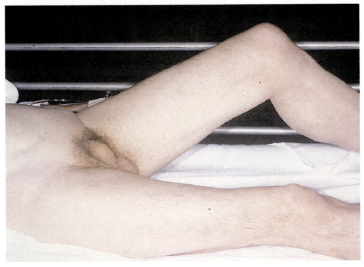

Fig. 92 Flexion of the hip in a patient with a psoas abscess.

20 / **Umbilicus**

Exomphalos

This is a rare condition presenting at birth. The abdominal wall fails to close about the umbilicus, leaving a variable amount of intestine and liver outside the abdominal cavity covered by amnion and peritoneum (Fig. 93). Associated gastrointestinal and other abnormalities are common.

Congenital umbilical hernia

A small defect is left at the site of the umbilicus (Fig. 94) but usually closes by the age of 2 years, so repair is seldom done before that age. Congenital umbilical hernias are commoner in Negro infants.

Acquired para-umbilical hernia

In adults hernias occur just above or below the umbilicus (Fig. 95). They are commoner with advancing age and obesity. The neck is often relatively small and strangulation is a danger. Such hernias are frequently irreducible because omentum becomes adherent within the sac. Repair is by the Mayo technique, overlapping the abdominal wall layers transversely over the defect.

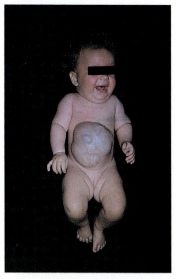

Fig. 93 Exomphalos in an infant.

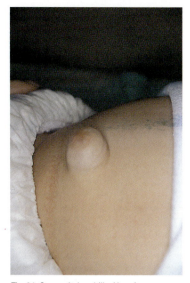

Fig. 94 Congenital umbilical hernia.

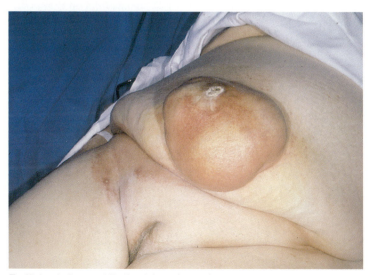

Fig. 95 Acquired para-umbilical hernia in an obese patient.

Umbilical sinuses and fistulae

Failure of the vitellointestinal duct or urachus to become obliterated are rare causes of discharge from the umbilicus (Fig. 96). The vitellointestinal duct connects the umbilicus to distal ileum and if it remains patent throughout its length intestinal contents will discharge, while a patent urachus connecting with the bladder will give a urinary fistula. Either duct may remain patent only at the umbilical end to form a blind sinus which discharges mucus. Persistence of the vitellointestinal duct at its end remote from the umbilicus results in Meckel's diverticulum.

Any kind of intra-abdominal sepsis may rarely discharge at the umbilicus.

Malignant nodule

Secondary carcinoma at the umbilicus (Sister Joseph's nodule, Fig. 97) presents as a hard nubbin. This is usually associated with an intra-abdominal primary such as carcinoma of the stomach, colon or ovary. Very occasionally secondary carcinoma from other sites such as the breast may appear at the umbilicus as a result of lymphatic spread. A secondary deposit at the umbilicus is usually associated with advanced cancer.

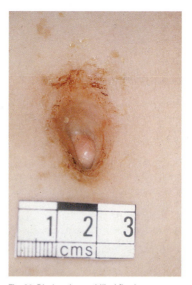

Fig. 96 Discharging umbilical fistula.

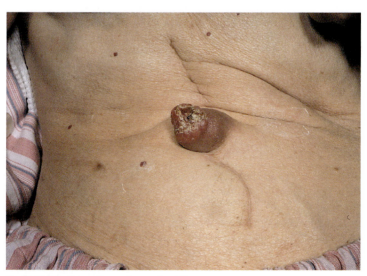

Fig. 97 Nodule of secondary carcinoma at umbilicus.

21 / **Hernia**

Epigastric hernia (Fig. 98)

These hernias are common, and often unnoticed. They occur through a small defect in the linea alba above the umbilicus. They should be differentiated from generalized divarication of the recti.

Clinical features   Usually only a small nubbin of omentum protrudes, which may be visible in the thin patient, but is often more easily detected by palpation. These little hernias are often tender and sometimes the patient gets pain on lying supine. Always consider an epigastric hernia in cases of localized epigastric pain.

Treatment   An epigastric hernia is treated by surgical repair of the defect.

Incisional hernia

Incisional hernias are common. They occur due to breakdown of the muscular and aponeurotic layers of an abdominal wound, often caused by wound infection, prolonged postoperative distension, or coughing. They are more frequent in vertical than transverse incisions, and in obese patients.

Clinical features   The hernia usually presents as a large bulge, due to diffuse weakness. Incisional hernias become more obvious when the supine patient actively raises his lower limbs or head from the couch, so tensing the abdominal muscles (Figs 99 & 100).

Incisional hernias with a narrow neck may strangulate. Strangulation can also occur in a loculus of a large hernia. The other important complication is intestinal obstruction, which may be subacute.

Treatment   An abdominal belt may give palliation for a large abdominal hernia. Repair can be complicated (for example requiring a synthetic mesh) and obese patients must diet first.

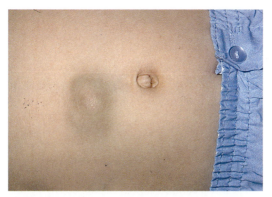

Fig. 98 This epigastric hernia is slightly displaced from the midline and shows well because of atypical skin discoloration.

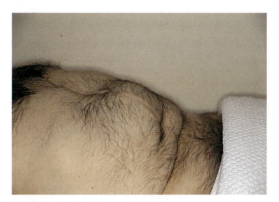

Fig. 99 Incisional hernia in lower midline scar.

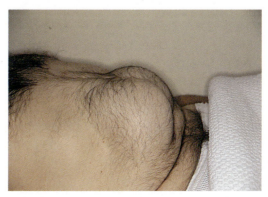

Fig. 100 Same patient as in Figure 99, with legs actively raised.

Inguinal hernia

Inguinal hernias are common and present as a lump in the groin which may cause aching and discomfort (Fig. 101).

Clinical types

Indirect inguinal hernia: consists of a peritoneal sac within the layers of the spermatic cord which can enlarge downwards into the scrotum (Fig. 102).

Direct hernia: consists of simple bulging of the peritoneum through a deficient posterior wall of the inguinal canal.

On examination an indirect hernia may be controlled by pressure of a finger over the internal inguinal ring.

Clinical features

Inguinal hernias may reduce spontaneously when the patient lies down or after gentle manipulation. If the patient then coughs the contents of the hernial sac may be seen to appear as a bulge and certainly felt with the flat of the hand. It may be necessary to stand the patient up to detect a small hernia. Large hernias may be difficult or impossible to reduce.

Treatment

Operation is the treatment of choice for most inguinal hernias and can be done under general or local anaesthetic.

Strangulation

If a hernia strangulates it becomes tense, tender, irreducible, and transmits no impulse on coughing. This requires emergency operation to save the contents from infarction.

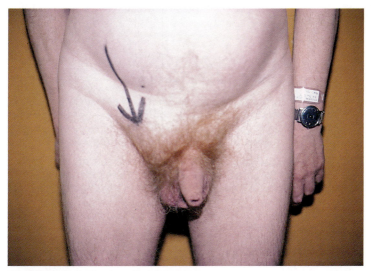

Fig. 101 Right inguinal hernia confined to the groin.

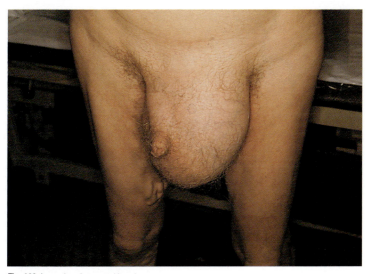

Fig. 102 Large inguinoscrotal hernia.

Congenital inguinal hernia

A congenital inguinal hernia resuts from failure of the processus vaginalis to obliterate. Lesser degrees of patent processus produce a hydrocele (fluid only, rather than abdominal contents transversing the processus).

Clinical features   A 'congenital hernia' may present at birth or a hernia may appear later in infancy or in childhood. The swelling may fill the scrotum or simply present in the groin (Fig. 103). Crying makes the hernia tense and prominent. Congenital hernias are commoner in boys than girls.

Femoral hernia

Femoral hernias are less common than inguinal hernias. They are more common in women than men.

Clinical features   A femoral hernia emerges through the femoral ring *below and lateral to the public tubercle* (while an inguinal hernia emerges above and medial to the tubercle). It is essential to use this rule, especially in the obese patient. The femoral ring is small and unyielding, so femoral hernias have a particular tendancy to become irreducible, causing strangulation or obstruction of the bowel. An elderly woman with small bowel obstruction should always be examined very carefully for a femoral hernia (Fig. 104), which is easy to miss. Sometimes only part of the bowel circumference is strangulated (Richter's hernia) so strangulation of the wall can occur without signs of obstruction.

Treatment   Because of their tendency to complications femoral hernias should always be repaired.

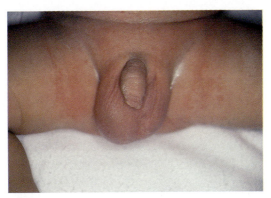

Fig. 103 Inguinal hernia in an infant filling the right scrotum.

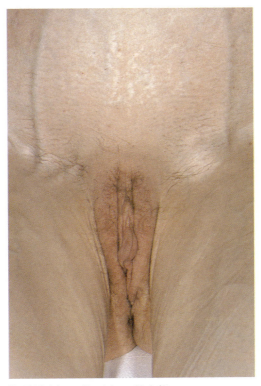

Fig. 104 Left femoral hernia in an elderly woman.

22 / **Groin**

Saphena varix   A prominent bulge of the upper long saphenous vein in the groin, just distal to an incompetent saphenofemoral valve, is caused by the high pressure of venous blood in the upright posture (Fig. 105). The bulge disappears when the patient lies down. A saphena varix is soft, compressible, and gives a thrill on coughing. It is usually associated with obvious varicose veins of the long saphenous system in the thigh and leg.

Inguinal   These nodes drain lymph from the lower limb,
lymphadenopathy   abdominal wall, back, perineum, and lower anal canal. Palpable lymph nodes in the groin are common due to forgotten trauma and infections of the legs. Significant lymphadenopathy (nodes larger than about 1.5 cm) usually affects several nodes. Their shape and distribution are characteristic (Fig. 106).

A single node may sometimes cause difficulty (e.g. Cloquet's node in the femoral canal can be difficult to distinguish from a femoral hernia). Whenever enlarged nodes are found, examine other lymph node areas, and the liver and spleen. Venereal diseases are specific causes for groin lymphadenopathy (syphilis, lymphogranuloma venereum, chancroid, gonorrhoea, HIV). Non-venereal infections and neoplasia are commoner in surgical practice. Remember cat scratch disease, which can cause impressive local lymphadenopathy. Occasionally infected lymph nodes can suppurate producing a groin abscess (Fig. 107).

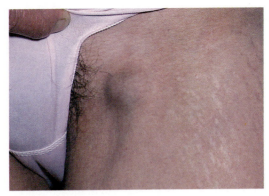

Fig. 105 Saphena varix.

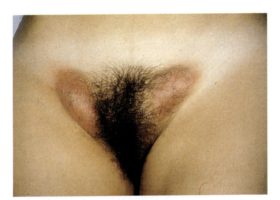

Fig. 106 Inguinal nodes.

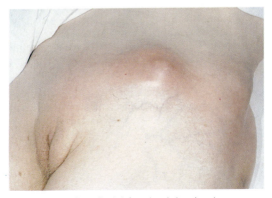

Fig. 107 Abscess formation in infected groin lymph nodes.

23 / Scrotum

Torsion of testis

Torsion of testis affects children and young adults. Predisposing factors are:

- horizontal testis
- high investment of the tunica vaginalis
- a persistent mesorchium
- testicular maldescent.

Clinical features Torsion gives sudden pain in the scrotum or lower abdomen. The testis lies high in the scrotum, is tender, and often swollen (Fig. 108). The scrotum can become inflamed and red. Children may vomit and the infant will simply scream and cry.

Differential diagnosis Differential diagnosis is from epididymo-orchitis and torsion of a testicular appendage. In the young child differentiate acute idiopathic scrotal oedema. This is rare and presents as sudden redness and oedema of the whole scrotum.

Treatment Immediate exploration is needed to prevent gangrene of the testis (Fig. 109) and both testes are fixed surgically (orchidopexy).

Torsion of testicular appendage

Torsion affects the appendix epididymis or appendix testis (hydatid of Morgagni, Fig. 110).

Clinical features Symptoms are similar to testicular torsion, but the pain tends to be less and the patient can usually walk about. Careful examination will localize the tenderness to one pole of the testis and the tender, swollen nubbin of the twisted appendage will be felt, and occasionally seen through the skin as a small bluish lump.

Treatment This condition will resolve spontaneously, but surgical exploration excludes testicular torsion and allows excision of the twisted appendage.

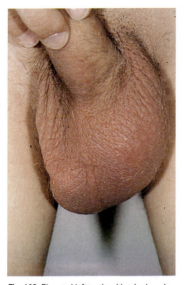

Fig. 108 Elevated left testis with a hydrocele in acute torsion.

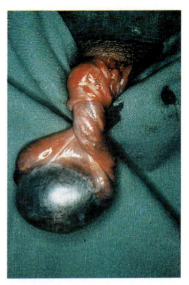

Fig. 109 Torsion of the testis with gangrene at operation.

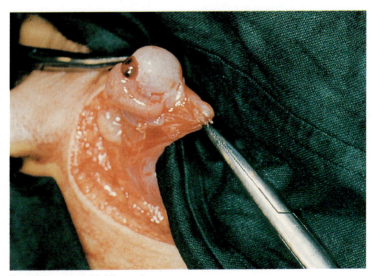

Fig. 110 Torted hydatid of Morgagni.

Hydrocele

A hydrocele is a collection of fluid within the tunica vaginalis around the testis.

Aetiology

In infants and children a hydrocele is associated with a patent processus vaginalis and is cured by ligating the processus.

In adults most hydroceles are seen in the middle-aged and elderly with no underlying cause (primary hydrocele, Fig. 111). In the younger adult they may result from inflammation, trauma, or tumour of the testis (secondary hydrocele).

Differential diagnosis

When examining the patient first be sure that the swelling is truly scrotal ('Can I get above it?', Fig. 112) rather than an inguinoscrotal hernia. Next ask, 'Can I readily feel the testis separate from the swelling?'. If so it may be an epididymal cyst: a hydrocele surrounds the testis which is difficult to palpate separately. Transillumination (Fig. 113) shows that the hydrocele contains clear fluid (Fig. 114) and reveals the position of the testis prior to aspiration of fluid.

Treatment

Aspiration of fluid may be followed by injection of sclerosant on one or more occasions as a form of treatment. Operation is a more certain method of cure and is indicated for a large or inconvenient hydrocele.

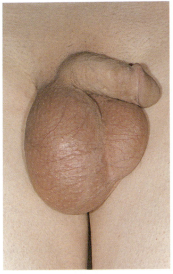

Fig. 111 Primary hydrocele.

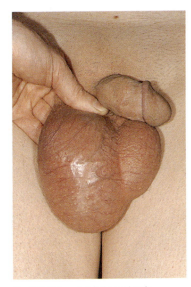

Fig. 112 Differentiating from a hernia.

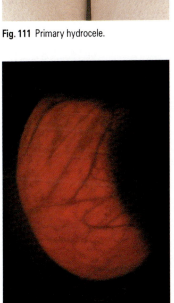

Fig. 113 Transillumination.

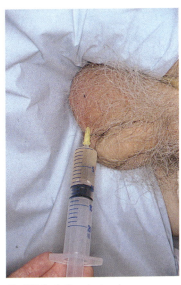

Fig. 114 Aspirating a hydrocele.

Testicular tumours

Clinical features
Testicular tumours present as a painless firm enlargement of the testis, most commonly in men aged between 18 and 40 years (Fig. 115). Only 15% will complain of pain and 10% will have an associated hydrocele. Lymphatic spread of testicular tumours is to the para-aortic nodes (not the groin), and the abdomen must be examined. Occasionally hormonal changes may produce gynaecomastia (Fig. 116).

Investigations
Ultrasound of the scrotum is useful for establishing the diagnosis. However, all young men with a firm testicular mass warrant surgical exploration. Additional investigation should include serum tumour markers and CT scanning to detect metastases.

Treatment
Treatment consists of orchidectomy by an inguinal approach. This is followed by a combination of radiotherapy and/or chemotherapy. The exact protocols depend on whether the tumour is a seminoma or a teratoma.

Prognosis
Cure rates have improved markedly. 5-year survival now exceeds 70% even in the presence of distant metastases.

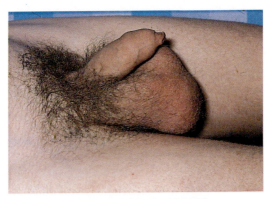

Fig. 115 Enlarged firm swelling within the right testicle.

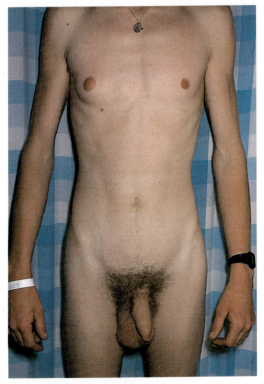

Fig. 116 The right testicle is enlarged and hanging low; there is associated bilateral gynaecomastia.

Cryptorchidism

The testes arise intra-abdominally and descend into the scrotum during the 7th month of intra-uterine life. Scrotal development and palpable testes should be present at birth. Failure of the testicle to reach the scrotum (Fig. 117) can lead to infertility and an increased risk of testicular malignancy.

Aetiology

The absence of one or both testes from the scrotum results from one of three situations:

True cryptorchidism: the testicle has stopped at any point during its descent. The majority, however, (80%) are palpable in the abdominal wall.

True anorchidism: rare.

Ectopia: the testicle has migrated to an abnormal site.

Differential diagnosis

Retractile testes are common due to an active cremasteric reflex. It may be impossible to differentiate this normal event from maldescent. With the patient relaxed an attempt is made to milk the testes into the scrotum.

Treatment

Treatment of undescended testes is by orchidopexy. The testis is mobilized by an inguinal approach and fixed in the scrotum. If the problem is discovered in later life, or testicular atrophy is present, then orchidectomy is preferred. True intra-abdominal testicles have a high risk of malignancy and should be removed.

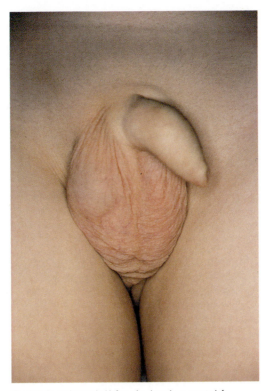

Fig. 117 An undescended left testis: there is an empty left hemiscrotum.

24 / Penis

Ulcers

An ulcerating lesion on the penis may arise for infective or neoplastic reasons.

Differential diagnosis

The differential diagnosis of infection includes syphilis, syphilitic chancre (Fig. 118), soft chancre (*Haemophilus* sp. infection) and condyloma. The important differential is from carcinoma, and diagnosis will often require a biopsy, particularly in the older patient.

Ulcerating carcinoma

Carcinoma of the penis (Fig. 119) is uncommon, affecting only 1 in 100 000 males, and very rare in the circumcised male. It arises most commonly after the age of 60 years and is rare under 45 years of age. Inadequate hygiene and herpes viruses are likely factors in the pathogenesis. The tumour is usually a low grade squamous cell carcinoma which spreads to the inguinal nodes.

Treatment

Early lesions can be treated by radiotherapy; more extensive tumours require some form of penile amputation. The prognosis in the absence of distant metastases is good.

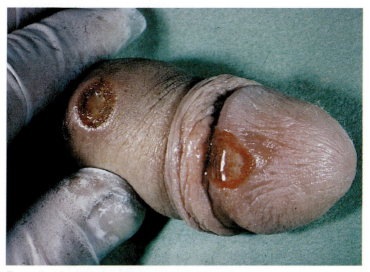

Fig. 118 Syphilitic chancres on the glans and shaft of the penis.

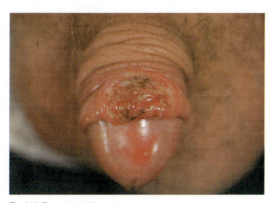

Fig. 119 The retracted foreskin reveals an ulcerating carcinoma.

Phimosis

At birth the prepuce is normally adherent to the glans and therefore non-retractile. By the end of the first year it can be fully retracted in most boys; for a few this process is delayed until they reach 3 or 4 years of age. Should infection occur behind the prepuce it may result in scarring, fibrosis of the prepuce, with consequent narrowing of the orifice; a phimosis (Fig. 120).

Treatment It is important, particularly in children, to distinguish a phimosis from a prepuce that has just never been retracted, which can be managed with advice. True phimosis is best treated by circumcision.

Paraphimosis

Paraphimosis occurs when a tight prepuce is retracted and fails to return. If it is not subsequently pushed back the constriction leads to swelling of the glans (Fig. 121), pain, and occasionally necrosis. It is this condition which must be avoided after male catheterization. It is the responsibility of the clinician to return the prepuce to its normal position.

Treatment The treatment of paraphimosis, if manual replacement is not possible, is by a dorsal slit or circumcision, which is urgently required.

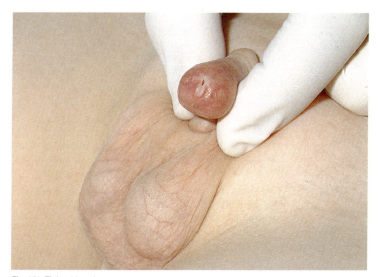

Fig. 120 Tight phimosis.

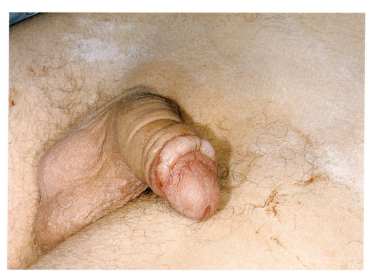

Fig. 121 A paraphimosis.

Epispadias

Epispadias is a rare congenital anomaly with the urethra opening on the dorsum of the penis (Fig. 122). The corpus spongiosum is usually deficient, and there is often an associated exstrophy of the bladder. Extensive defects may reach the bladder neck and be associated with urinary incontinence.

Treatment   Treatment involves reconstruction of the urethra and bladder neck. In some cases urinary diversion may be required to achieve continence.

Hypospadias

Hypospadias is the commonest urethral anomaly in boys (approximately 1 in 300 births). It results from failure of fusion of the urethral folds on the ventral surface of the genital tubercle. The opening of the meatus is proximally displaced on the shaft of the penis (Fig. 123).

Treatment   The majority (85%) have a glandular or coronal defect which is repaired only for cosmetic reasons. The remainder can be corrected by one-stage surgical procedures before the boys reach school age.

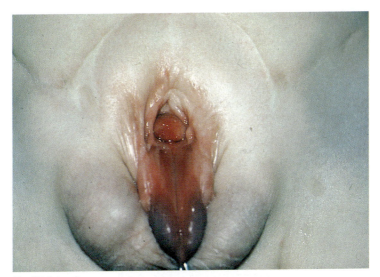

Fig. 122 Epispadias.

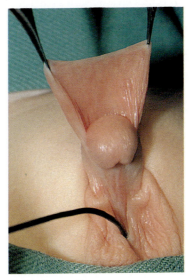

Fig. 123 Hypospadias.

Priapism

This is an uncommon disorder where there is a prominent painful erection of both corpora cavernosa, with the corpus spongiosum and glans unaffected (Fig. 124).

Aetiology The erection appears to result from sludging of blood in the sinuses of the corpora cavernosa, but the reason for this remains unknown. It is associated with patients on renal dialysis, sickle cell disease and leukaemia.

Treatment Urgent treatment is required to relieve the priapism. Delay will increase the risk of fibrosis and the chance of subsequent impotence.

Aspiration techniques are usually ineffective. The first option is the use of a biopsy needle to create a fistula between the flaccid glans and the corpora cavernosa. If this is unsuccessful then a saphenocorporal shunt will be required. If treatment is delayed beyond 12 hours the risk of impotence is high.

Fractured penis

Injury to the erect penis can cause a rupture of the corpora cavernosa; a fractured penis. The erection will dissipate and bruising will occur (Fig. 125).

Treatment The patient is most likely to be impotent and primary repair of the defect is the best therapeutic option.

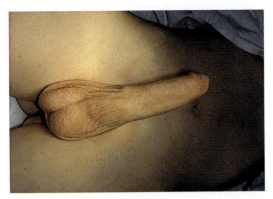

Fig. 124 Priapism: note the flaccid glans.

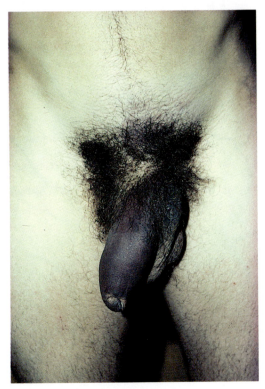

Fig. 125 Bruising from a fractured penis.

25 / Anus

Fissure

This is a mucosal tear lying within the anal canal: it is an acutely painful condition. Most fissures arise in the midline either anteriorly or posteriorly (Fig. 126). Once established, a cycle of constipation, tearing and pain prolongs the condition. Some cases are secondary to inflammatory bowel disease (see p. 107). The ends of the tear become swollen and enlarged with the development of a hypertrophic papilla internally. Externally a fibrotic skin tag develops which is known as a sentinel pile (Fig. 127).

Clinical features   The classical history is of painful defaecation with bright red rectal bleeding. The pain often continues after a bowel movement delaying the next defaecation and changing the regular bowel habit. Gentle examination will reveal a sentinel pile and the fissure. If surgery is inevitable further examination is more kindly performed under anaesthesia. Then it must include both sigmoidoscopy and proctoscopy.

Treatment   Early cases can be treated by relieving the constipation with dietary advice and laxatives. Most require surgical treatment either by manual dilatation or sphincterotomy. Whilst the former is simpler it may occasionally cause major sphincter damage so that sphincterotomy is preferable.

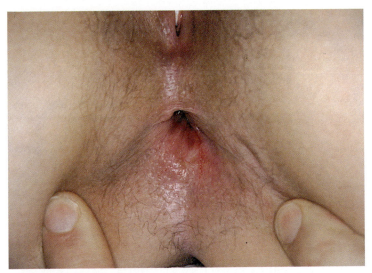

Fig. 126 An early posterior anal fissure.

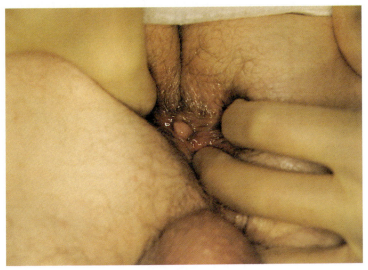

Fig. 127 A chronic anal fissure with a sentinel pile.

Fistula

Fistula development is most commonly secondary to an earlier abscess which has spontaneously burst or been surgically drained.

Clinical features The fistula produces a chronic purulent discharge from the external orifice with associated pruritus ani and staining of the underclothes. On examination a discharging orifice may be obvious. Digital palpation will often reveal a track, which can also be cannulated with a probe (Fig. 128). This latter manoeuvre is usually only performed under general anaesthesia. The internal orifice arises from one of the anal glands. Goodsall's rule states that fistulae anterior to the coronal plane usually have a straight track. Those behind the anus will commonly have the internal opening in the midline and pursue a more tortuous course.

Other causes of fistula in the perianal region include Crohn's disease, radiation, trauma and neoplasm. All fistula walls should be biopsied.

Treatment Treatment is almost always surgical and consists of laying open the fistulous track. If the track crosses the sphincter more specialized procedures are required to preserve continence (Fig. 129).

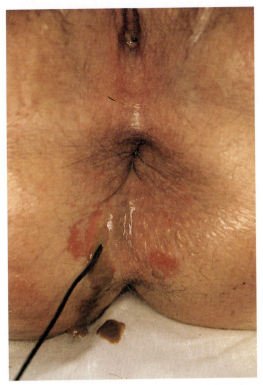

Fig. 128 A perianal fistula in the 7 o'clock position with the probe running to the midline posteriorly.

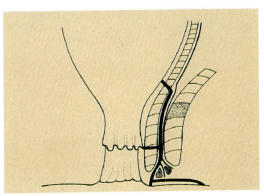

Fig. 129 A diagram of the tracks that perianal fistulae may follow.

Prolapse

Clinical features

The patient presents complaining of a mass presenting at the anus. Initially the mass is small and only occurs on straining. The size of the prolapse increases with time. It is important to distinguish this condition from haemorrhoids which are essentially a form of mucosal prolapse. In true rectal prolapse the full thickness of the bowel wall descends through the anus (Fig. 130).

As the prolapse progresses it descends whenever the patient stands up. The resulting discomfort and hygiene problems are extremely distressing. The prolapsed bowel secretes mucus which irritates and the easily damaged bowel bleeds on contact. As the anal sphincter is stretched then faecal incontinence ensues.

On examination the prolapse may not initially be apparent. The patient must be asked to strain and may need to do so in a squatting position. Digital examination will reveal a lax anal sphincter that cannot contract forcibly.

Investigations

Sigmoidoscopy is essential. Occasionally it will reveal a polypoid tumour which has been prolapsing peranally (Fig. 131).

Treatment

Treatment is surgical and a variety of procedures are available. No one procedure suits all patients. Treatment of the prolapse may be effective, but incontinence may remain a problem.

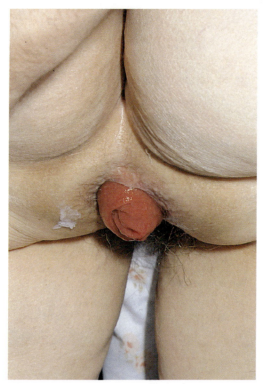

Fig. 130 A full thickness rectal prolapse: the mucosa is moist and pink.

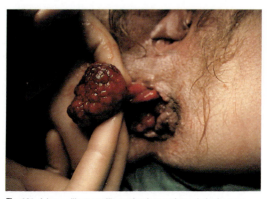

Fig. 131 A large villous papilloma that has prolapsed via the anus.

Perianal abscess

A perianal abscess is a common surgical emergency with a higher incidence in men. The abscess is thought to arise in the anal glands which lie in the intersphincteric plane. If the pus tracks inferiorly a perianal abscess presents externally. The pus may also track superiorly to develop as a supralevator abscess or laterally to form an ischiorectal abscess.

Clinical features Superficial abscesses produce the most pain, which is often related to sitting or moving. They are clinically obvious on external examination. The deeper abscesses may expand without causing much pain, but produce symptoms of systemic sepsis. Rectal examination reveals a tender swelling (Fig. 132) which may be clearer after a bimanual examination.

Treatment Treatment is by incision and drainage: internally into the rectum if the abscess is within the external sphincter; otherwise externally. Patients must be warned that a fistula may result.

Pilonidal sinus (Fig. 133)

Most probably, this is an acquired sinus secondary to trapping of hair in the sacrococcygeal area. Pilonidal sinuses are therefore more common after puberty in men and women with an abundance of hair.

Clinical features The sinus is usually asymptomatic until it becomes infected and an abscess results. Pain and tenderness in the natal cleft reveal the lesion. Hair may be seen protruding from the openings.

Treatment Treatment is by surgical incision and drainage. Keeping the natal cleft free of hair will reduce the chance of recurrence.

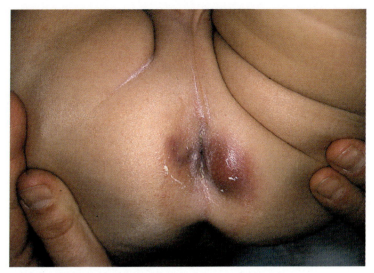

Fig. 132 A perianal abscess in an infant.

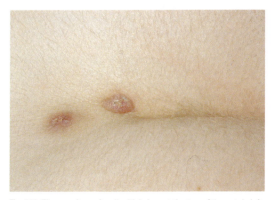

Fig. 133 The openings of a pilonidal sinus at the top of the natal cleft.

Haemorrhoids

Haemorrhoids are present in all adults; they are vascular cushions normally sited at the 3, 7 and 11 o'clock positions and contribute to continence. They only require treatment if they become symptomatic.

Aetiology

The commonest cause of symptomatic haemorrhoids is constipation and straining at stool; aggravating factors include obesity and pregnancy.

Clinical features

Patients will complain of 'piles' to describe a variety of symptoms. It is important to take an accurate history and determine the specific nature of the complaint. Severe pain is not a feature of haemorrhoids unless they have prolapsed and become thrombosed. The earliest symptom is bleeding, which is bright red and separate from the stool (first degree). As they progress they may prolapse through the anus on straining (second degree, Fig. 134). At a later stage the prolapse may require manual replacement or become fixed (third degree, Fig. 135).

First degree haemorrhoids are only visible on proctoscopy. The other degrees can be seen on visual examination of the perineum as the patient is requested to strain. Digital examination cannot feel internal haemorrhoids. In the absence of thrombosis, pain during the examination should raise the possibility of a fissure.

Treatment

Treatment must include dietary advice and the management of constipation. First and second degree haemorrhoids will respond to injection sclerotherapy and band ligation. Third degree haemorrhoids will usually require haemorrhoidectomy.

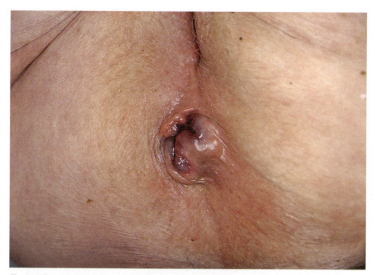

Fig. 134 Second degree haemorrhoids produced on straining.

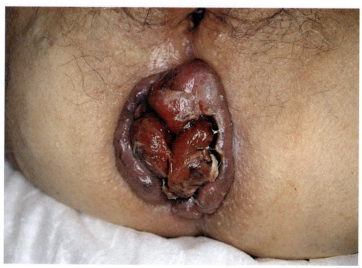

Fig. 135 Large prolapsed and thrombosed third degree haemorrhoids.

Carcinoma

Whereas carcinoma of the rectum is a common disease that of the anus is rare. Indeed half of the lesions presenting at the anus are probably spreading low rectal tumours. Anal carcinomas are of squamous cell origin.

Clinical features   The major complaint is of a lump at the anus or bleeding due to 'piles'. There is often a discharge and discomfort. On examination a nodular ulcerating lesion is obvious at the anal verge (Fig. 136). Digital palpation of the rectal canal and vagina will reveal the extent of the disease. Spread will occur via the inguinal glands which should be examined carefully. Diagnosis can be made on biopsy; the tumour lies below the mucocutaneous junction so that anaesthesia is required.

Treatment   Treatment is a combination of radiotherapy, chemotherapy and surgery.

Crohn's disease

This chronic granulomatous inflammatory disease most commonly affects the terminal ileum. Although separated by apparently normal bowel, complex fissures, fistulae (Figs 137 & 138) and abscesses of the anus are seen in up to 25% of patients.

Clinical features   The patient presents with the typical features of Crohn's disease; abdominal pain, diarrhoea and constitutional upset. Inspection reveals the anal findings which may be strangely asymptomatic. Biopsy of the anorectal lesion will often give the diagnosis.

Treatment   Treatment is that of the primary disease. The anal lesions will often resolve, but if symptomatic should be treated on merit.

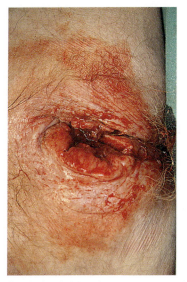

Fig. 136 A typical ulcerating squamous carcinoma of the anus.

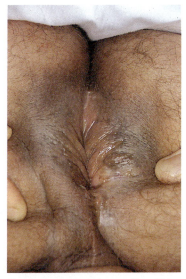

Fig. 137 A typical Crohn's anus with multiple weeping fistulae.

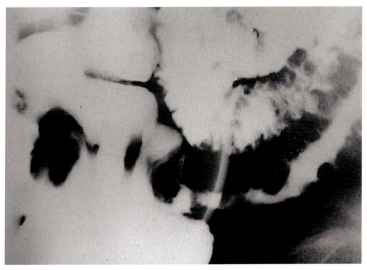

Fig. 138 A barium follow-through demonstrating Crohn's disease of the terminal ileum: rose-thorn ulcers are evident as well as a string sign caused by intestinal stenosis.

26 / Stomata

Tracheostomy

Direct access to the trachea via the neck may be temporary to provide airway support, or permanent following laryngectomy. The following types of access are employed.

Mini-tracheotomy

A small tube is inserted through the cricopharyngeal membrane under local anaesthesia. Its main use is to permit tracheobronchial suction.

Temporary tracheostomy

A temporary tracheostomy is still required for some patients who require long-term ventilatory support. It has many advantages over endotracheal intubation such as:

- patient comfort
- reduced dead space
- easier suction of mouth and trachea
- protection from aspiration
- reduced chance of laryngeal damage.

Initially a cuffed tube will be inserted (Fig. 139). However, many patients can then cope with a valved tube, which enables them to talk normally (Fig. 140).

Permanent tracheostomy

A single end opening in the neck is needed after laryngectomy. Patients eventually wear a gauze filter to reduce particulate inhalation and many learn to speak using swallowed air.

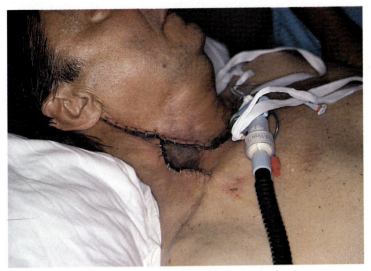

Fig. 139 Patient with a cuffed tracheostomy tube in place on a ventilator.

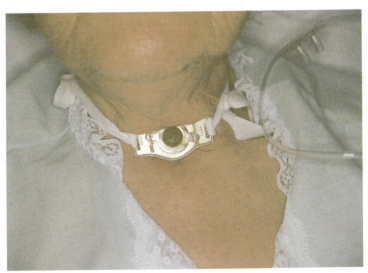

Fig. 140 A silver valved tracheostomy tube that allows the patient to speak.

Colostomy

A colostomy is an opening of the colon on to the skin. The discharge from a colostomy is solid or semi-solid and the bowel is joined flush to the skin. Two basic types are commonly performed.

End colostomy

An end colostomy is a single end after an abdominoperineal resection or Hartmann's procedure. These are performed in the left iliac fossa and frequently shrink to become only 1 or 2 cm across (Fig. 141).

Loop colostomy

Loop colostomies are performed after difficult anastomotic surgery to permit healing without a faecal stream. Both proximal and distal ends open into the colostomy bag. The bowel is initially held up by a bar under the central bridge (Fig. 142); this is removed after 7 days and the gut shrinks back to a reasonable size. Most loop colostomies are performed in the right upper quadrant. They can be closed after the distal anastomosis has healed; usually after 6–8 weeks.

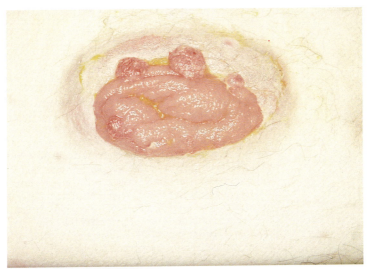

Fig. 141 An established end colostomy in the left iliac fossa.

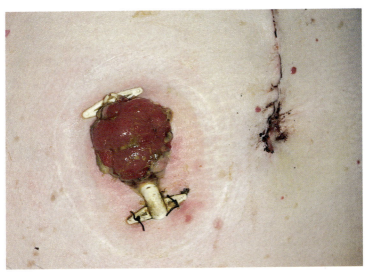

Fig. 142 A recently formed transverse loop defunctioning colostomy with the bridge still in place.

Ileostomy

Some patients with inflammatory bowel disease require complete resection of the colon and rectum. The ileum must then be brought out as a terminal stoma in the right iliac fossa. Ileal contents are fluid and contain active proteolytic enzymes which are normally denatured by the caecal bacteria. For this reason they must be kept off the skin which would otherwise become very sore. An ileostomy does not therefore end flush with the skin, but requires a spout of 3–5 cm (Fig. 143). This directs the discharge into the bag and preserves the skin. Ileostomies, unlike colostomies, discharge continuously and the appliance must be worn at all times.

Urostomy

A similar terminal arrangement is required if it becomes necessary to remove the bladder. Ureters cannot be anastomosed directly to skin as the orifice would stenose and obstruct. They are therefore drained into an isolated segment of ileum which is brought out as a spout—an ileal conduit. (Fig. 144). In this case urine needs to be kept off the skin to avoid a 'nappy' rash which can be severe.

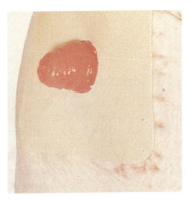

Fig. 143 The protruding spout of an ileostomy.

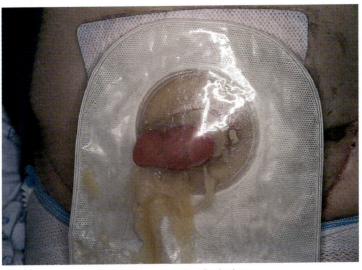

Fig. 144 A urostomy with the spout lying within the collecting bag.

Acute ischaemia

Aetiology Embolism is the commonest cause of acute ischaemia, often from the heart in atrial fibrillation or after myocardial infarction. Another important cause is thrombosis affecting the arteries in a limb with pre-existing arterial disease. Trauma is another cause of acute ischaemia and arterial injury should always be considered in cases of penetrating wounds or fractures near major arteries (Fig. 145).

Clinical features Classical acute ischaemia produces the six p's:
- pain
- pallor
- paraesthesiae
- pulselessness
- paralysis
- perishing cold.

Swelling is not a feature of acute ischaemia but may occur if there is secondary venous thrombosis.

Prognosis In assessing an acutely ischaemic foot (Fig. 147), sensory loss is a critical sign, which means that the extremity will be lost unless blood flow can be rapidly restored. Muscle paralysis is a late sign, while 'fixed staining' of the skin (Fig. 148) indicates a situation beyond salvage.

In 'acute on chronic ischaemia' some blood flow is preserved through established collaterals and the foot may therefore remain viable.

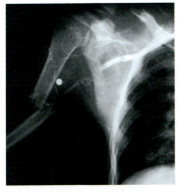

Fig. 145 Arteriogram showing brachial artery damage by fractured humerus.

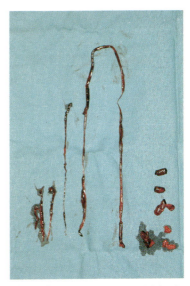

Fig. 146 Platelet thrombus (bottom right) and propagated clot extracted at embolectomy.

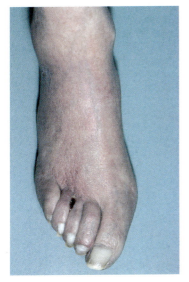

Fig. 147 Acutely ischaemic foot.

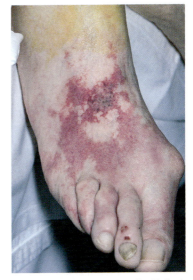

Fig. 148 Neglected acute ischaemia with fixed staining of the skin.

Chronic ischaemia

Only a small proportion of patients with arterial disease causing intermittent claudication go on to develop limb-threatening ischaemia. *Ischaemic rest pain* usually affects the toes and forefoot. It is worse at night and the patient may hang the foot out of bed, walk about, or sleep sitting upright in a chair to lessen the pain.

Clinical features

A chronically ischaemic foot may look pale or show the rubor of cutaneous vasodilatation ('pre-gangrene', Fig. 149). Classical signs of chronic ischaemia include slow capillary refilling (Figs 150 & 151), pallor on elevating the limb (perhaps with venous guttering), and sometimes marked rubor and cyanosis in the dependent foot after elevating the limb (a positive Buerger's test). Hair loss is a nonspecific and unhelpful sign.

Investigations

Pulse palpation. Absent femoral or popliteal pulses are important, but impalpable foot pulses are of little help in evaluation.

Doppler systolic pressure measurement. Measurement at ankle level provides simple objective evidence of ischaemia and its severity. Ankle pressure index is ankle pressure divided by brachial pressure (normal $\geqslant$ 1.0). 'Critical ischaemia' is a specific term used when the ankle pressure is less than 50 mmHg.

Punctate ischaemia

Small ischaemic patches on the toes suggest small emboli or vasculitis as a cause.

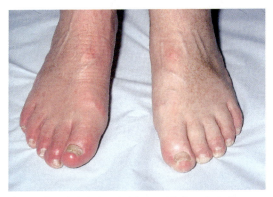

Fig. 149 Chronically ischaemic right foot with dependent rubor.

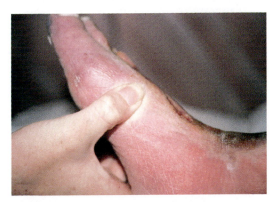

Fig. 150 Applying firm pressure to test capillary return.

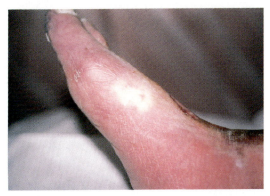

Fig. 151 Same foot as in Figure 150, showing delayed capillary return.

Chronic ischaemia (contd)

Trophic changes

Ulcers or gangrene (trophic lesions) develop either spontaneously or as a result of injury, such as friction from footwear or damage during chiropody.

Clinical features

Small ulcers often start between the toes (Fig. 152) or on the heel (Fig. 153). These sites should always be examined. Ischaemic ulcers usually have a sloughy base and the edge may be gangrenous. There is usually little evidence of granulation tissue. Deep ischaemic ulcers may expose tendon or bone.

Before frank gangrene occurs the skin becomes cold and deeply discoloured (Fig. 154). These changes are most marked distally, on the toes and forefoot.

Differential diagnosis

Ulcers about the ankle are more often venous in origin, although they may be perpetuated by ischaemia. Vasculitic disorders such as rheumatoid arthritis should also be considered as causes of ulceration.

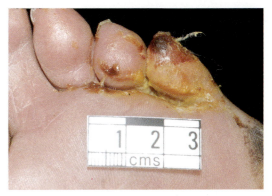

Fig. 152 Ulceration between the toes in an ischaemic foot.

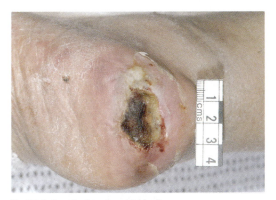

Fig. 153 Ischaemic ulceration of the heel.

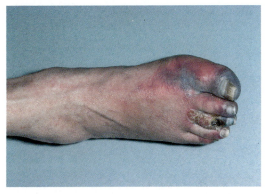

Fig. 154 Severely ischaemic foot with impending tissue loss.

28 / **Gangrene**

Dry gangrene

Dry gangrene occurs when dead tissue mummifies without infection (Fig. 155).

Clinical features   Toes are most commonly affected. The result is a dry, black digit with a sharp line of demarcation with healthy living tissue.

Treatment   Because it is painless and uninfected there is usually no indication to amputate a digit affected by dry gangrene which will eventually separate (spontaneous or auto-amputation).

Wet gangrene

In wet gangrene there is tissue necrosis with putrefaction. Clostridia are often involved.

Clinical features   The part is blackened and becomes foul smelling (Fig. 156). Because the dead tissue is in continuity with living tissue, toxins reach the circulation and make the patient unwell and confused.

Treatment   Debridement or amputation is mandatory to prevent the eventual outcome of septicaemia and death.

Local amputation of gangrenous toes or parts of the foot will only heal in the presence of adequate blood supply. If the whole foot is ischaemic due to occlusions of larger arteries then these must be dealt with, or a major amputation (below or even above the knee) will be required.

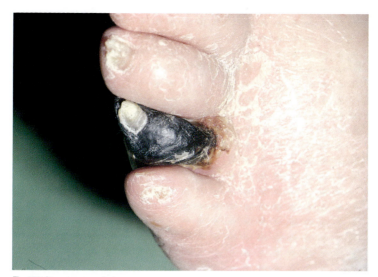

Fig. 155 Dry gangrene of a toe.

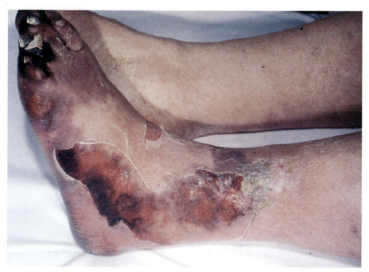

Fig. 156 Wet gangrene affecting the whole foot.

Ulcers, gangrene and foot infections are common in diabetics. Four factors predispose:

- Small vessel disease affecting arterioles in the foot and toes.
- Early onset of atherosclerosis in larger arteries, particularly those below the knee.
- Neuropathy causing diminished sensation with loss of reflexes. This allows ischaemic and infected lesions (Fig. 157) to develop without pain and Charcot's joints may occur.
- A tendency to development and rapid spread of infection.

Clinical features Necrosis often starts at points of pressure (e.g. under the metatarsal heads). Sinuses form which can track along tissue planes (Fig. 158). Small surface lesions often conceal deep infection in the diabetic foot. Radiographs show bony changes in the later stages. If contained pus is suspected, early drainage is essential.

Treatment Sometimes amputation of an infected or ischaemic toe will suffice but often pus has spread proximally along the web spaces and a *'ray' amputation* is required (Fig. 159). These amputations are left open to allow free drainage and will slowly heal provided the blood supply is adequate.

In assessing the blood supply to a diabetic foot remember that arterial calcification may give artefactually elevated Doppler systolic pressure readings

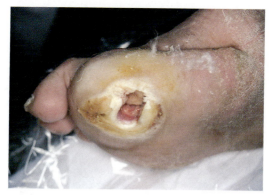

Fig. 157 Deep indolent ulcer in a diabetic foot.

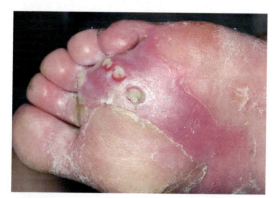

Fig. 158 Sinuses with infection tracking through the sole of a diabetic foot.

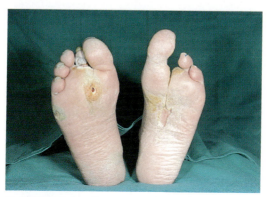

Fig. 159 Diabetic feet with a ray amputation on left and a neuropathic ulcer on right.

30 / **Aneurysm**

Aortic aneurysm Abdominal aortic aneurysms (Fig. 160) are common in older men and may rupture, causing sudden death, or presenting with abdominal and back pain, a pulsatile abdominal mass, and shock.

If detected before rupture these aneurysms can be grafted with low mortality. Some cause pain in the abdomen or back, or the patient may notice pulsation in his abdomen. More often they cause no symptoms.

Aortic aneurysms can be difficult to feel. The hand must be kept still to the left of the umbilicus. Size can be estimated using the fingers of both hands. An ultrasound scan confirms a diagnosis.

Femoral aneurysm A femoral aneurysm presents as a pulsatile lump in the groin (Fig. 161). True femoral aneurysms are uncommon but false aneurysm not infrequently follows aortobifemoral grafting.

Popliteal aneurysm Popliteal aneurysms most often cause symptoms by emboli (giving ischaemic toes) or by thrombosis (giving acute limb ischaemia). Rupture is uncommon.

The aneurysm presents as a pulsatile swelling behind the knee (Fig. 162) and should be suspected when the popliteal pulse feels unusually obvious. Pulsation distinguishes a popliteal aneurysm from a semimembranosus bursa or a popliteal (Baker's) cyst. Popliteal aneurysms are often bilateral and may be associated with abdominal aortic aneurysm.

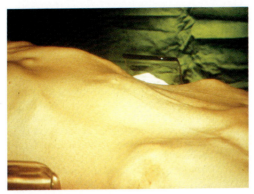

Fig. 160 Visible abdominal aortic aneurysm in a thin patient.

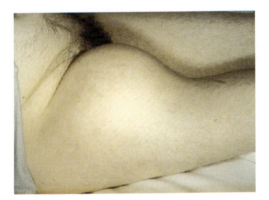

Fig. 161 Large right femoral aneurysm.

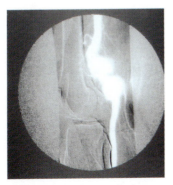

Fig. 162 Arteriogram showing a popliteal aneurysm.

31 / **Distal emboli**

Large emboli cause acute limb ischaemia, but small emboli reach the digital vessels, giving ischaemia or gangrene of individual digits (Fig. 163); or small ischaemic patches of skin. The important differential diagnosis is vasculitis with occlusion of small vessels.

Small emboli may originate from localized arterial stenoses (Fig. 164) where platelet thrombi can form, or from aneurysms (especially popliteal aneurysms).

'Trash foot' 'Trash foot' is the term used for ischaemia and gangrene of the toes following dislodgement of embolic material during surgery for aortic aneurysm (Fig. 165). Remember that emboli cannot pass to an extremity where there is already occlusion of a major limb artery.

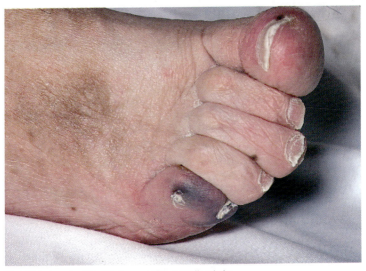

Fig. 163 Ischaemia of the little toe caused by a small embolus.

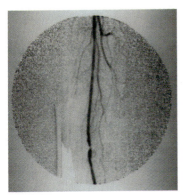

Fig. 164 Stenosis of superficial femoral artery giving rise to emboli.

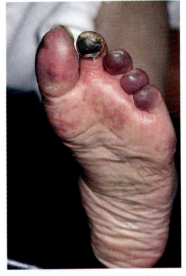

Fig. 165 'Trash foot' caused by embolic material.

32 / Raynaud's phenomenon

Definition   Episodic coldness and pallor of the fingers (or toes), usually precipitated by exposure to cold. On rewarming cyanosis and rubor occur. In severe progressive cases fingers are cold and painful even at room temperature, and occasionally distal gangrene occurs (Fig. 166).

Aetiology   Idiopathic Raynaud's disease is the commonest type, usually affecting women from teenage onwards. Some go on to develop connective tissue disorders such as scleroderma or rheumatoid. There are many other causes including vibration injury, arteriosclerosis, drugs (contraceptive pill, ergot, cytotoxics), and cold agglutinins or cryoglobulins in the blood. Unilateral Raynaud's syndrome in a man suggests the possibility of a localized lesion such as cervical rib (Fig. 167) causing thoracic outlet compression.

Raynaud's phenomenon may be caused by pure vasospasm of the digital arteries, or obstruction combined with vasospasm, and the latter in particular may affect single digits (Fig. 168).

Treatment   Treatment consists of measures to keep the hands warm and avoidance of smoking. Many drugs have been tried with inconsistent results. Sympathectomy often works well for lower limb vasospasm, but in the upper limbs the result is usually temporary.

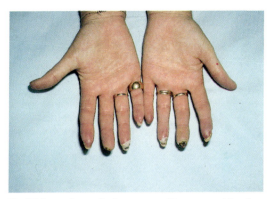

Fig. 166 Severe Raynaud's phenomenon with gangrene of tips of digits.

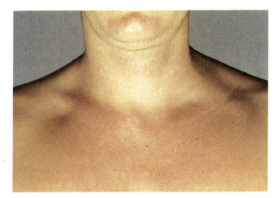

Fig. 167 Left cervical rib causing a bulge in the supraclavicular fossa.

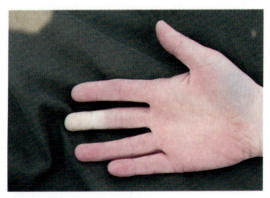

Fig. 168 Vasospasm of a single digit.

Varicose veins

Clinical features

These widened, elongated, tortuous veins become obvious when the patient stands, bulging under the skin and often causing cosmetic embarrassment. Other symptoms are heaviness, aching, and ankle swelling. Occasionally lipodermatosclerosis or ulcers may result.

There is often valvular incompetence between the deep veins and the superficial varicose veins which must be detected and dealt with if treatment is planned. Sites of incompetence are:

- the saphenofemoral junction in the groin
- a short saphenous termination behind the knee
- direct perforating veins low in the thigh or in the calf.

Investigations

Saphenofemoral incompetence may give a saphena varix (Fig. 169)—a groin lump which compresses easily, imparts a thrill on coughing and disappears on lying down. Incompetence is demonstrated by the Brodie–Trendelenburg test (Fig. 170). The sites of varicose veins are noted, the patient sits and the leg is elevated. The long saphenous vein is controlled by finger pressure in the groin or a venous tourniquet on the upper thigh. The patient stands. Incompetent perforating veins distal to the tourniquet give rapid refilling. Saphenofemoral incompetence causes rapid refilling of the veins from above when the tourniquet is removed.

Similar tourniquet tests can be done to determine the sites of more distal incompetent valves. All of this is more sensitively done using a Doppler probe to detect flow signals in the veins.

Percussion of veins with the finger shows which veins interconnect. A fluid thrill is transmitted to the fingers placed over connecting venous channels.

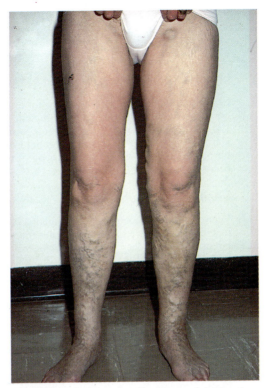

Fig. 169 Bilateral varicose veins with saphena varix in left groin.

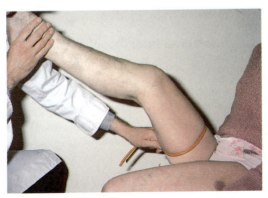

Fig. 170 Brodie–Trendelenburg test in the examination of varicose veins.

Lipodermatosclerosis (varicose eczema)

Clinical features Chronic venous hypertension in the skin results in liposclerosis, pigmentation, and eczematous change (Fig. 171). Sometimes whitish discolouration ('atrophie blanche') is seen. Oedema is common but eventually fibrosis may produce scarred tissue about the ankle with oedema above.

Venous ulceration

Venous ulcers are commoner in women. They may occur in a setting of severe superficial venous incompetence, but often there is deep venous incompetence, sometimes secondary to deep vein thrombosis. About a quarter of patients with 'venous' ulcers also have arterial disease which can delay healing and must be recognized.

Clinical features Ulceration may be precipitated by minor trauma. It often occurs in an area of florid lipodermatosclerosis although sometimes there is little surrounding skin change. Venous (or 'gravitational') ulcers occur typically near the medial or lateral malleolus and the 'gaiter' area above (Fig. 172). The ulcer base may contain smelly slough, or healthy granulation tissue, depending on the effectiveness of local care. Venous ulcers range from a few millimetres in diameter to circumferential ulceration. Pain is variable.

Superficial thrombophlebitis

Clinical features Superficial thrombophlebitis presents as a painful, tender, reddened area of skin (Fig. 173) overlying veins (usually varicose) in which tender thrombus may be palpable. It is not a cause of pulmonary embolism.

Treatment Treatment consists of anti-inflammatory and analgesic drugs, and perhaps a poultice.

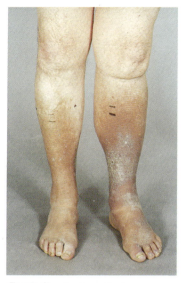

Fig. 171 Chronic venous skin changes.

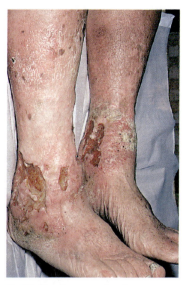

Fig. 172 Chronic venous ulceration.

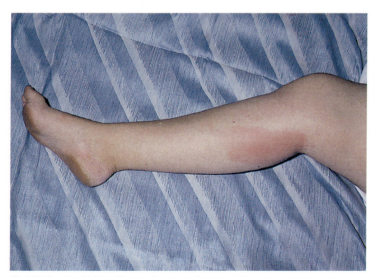

Fig. 173 Thrombophlebitis of long saphenous vein in upper calf.

Deep vein thrombosis

Deep vein thrombosis is commonest in the venous plexuses of the calf, particularly postoperatively. Other predisposing factors are pregnancy, the contraceptive pill, serious ill health and immobility.

Clinical features　Many deep vein thromboses cause no symptoms or signs. Swelling is the commonest sign (Fig. 174) and may occur below the knee only, or may affect the thigh as well in iliofemoral thrombosis. The presence and degree of swelling can be documented by measuring the circumference of the limb at a known distance from a bony point (e.g. tip of medial malleolus) and comparing this with the unaffected limb (Fig. 175). Mild oedema can be detected by the more turgid feel of the relaxed calf muscles when 'wobbled' between the fingers with the knee flexed.

Thrombosis in the deep veins may cause significant phlebitis which gives pain, tenderness, and occasionally redness. Tenderness is commonest in the midline of the calf. Homans' sign is pain in the calf muscles on sudden forced dorsiflexion of the ankle but should probably be abandoned.

Investigations　The diagnosis is supported by finding no signal in the femoral vein at the groin with a simple Doppler probe, or by failure to enhance any flow signal by squeezing the calf. Venography or duplex scanning confirm the diagnosis.

Venous gangrene

Venous gangrene is a rare condition that is usually associated with serious underlying disease such as malignancy.

Clinical features　Gross venous thrombosis causes capillary obstruction to produce a swollen, hot, and sometimes blistered limb with distal gangrene (Fig. 176). It is often a terminal event, but if the limb and the patient recover the amount of tissue loss may be surprisingly small.

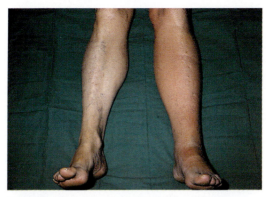

Fig. 174 Deep venous thrombosis of the left leg which appears swollen and discoloured.

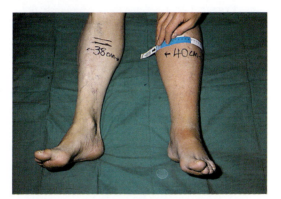

Fig. 175 The same patient as in Figure 174 demonstrating calf measurement at a fixed point below the tibial tubercle.

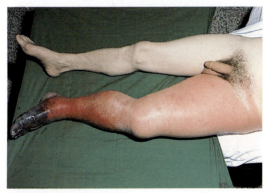

Fig. 176 Gross iliofemoral venous thrombosis which has led to venous gangrene of the forefoot.

34 / Lymphoedema

Aetiology Lymphoedema may be primary, or secondary, to infection (e.g. filariasis) or malignant disease and its treatment (surgery or radiotherapy) (Fig. 177). Impaired lymphatic drainage produces painless swelling of the limb. In the early stages this may be postural, but the oedema later becomes persistent and associated with tissue fibrosis, giving the classical 'non-pitting oedema' (Fig. 178). Remember that cardiac or venous oedema is much commoner than lymphoedema as a cause of leg swelling.

Primary lymphoedema

Clinical features Primary lymphoedema most commonly presents as unilateral ankle swelling in teenage women. The other leg is often involved later. Progression is slow. Lymphography (using contrast or radio-isotopes) shows obliteration of distal lymphatics.

Less common varieties are:

- rapidly developing unilateral lymphoedema at any age due to obliteration of proximal lymphatics and nodes
- true 'congenital' lymphoedema occurring soon after birth and associated with chylous collections and other abnormalities. Large incompetent lymphatic trunks are present. Familial congenital bilateral lymphoedema due to absent lymphatics is called Milroy's disease.

Complications Complications of lymphoedema are cellulitis, leakage of chyle, hyperkeratosis of the soles and very rarely lymphangiosarcoma (Fig. 179).

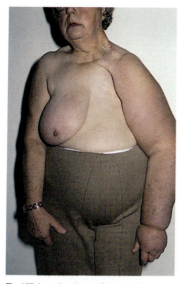

Fig. 177 Lymphoedema of the arm after mastectomy and radiotherapy.

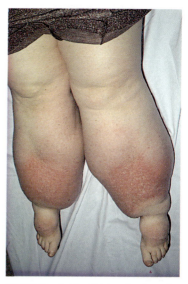

Fig. 178 Chronic idiopathic lymphoedema of lower limbs.

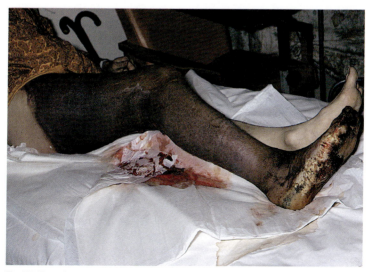

Fig. 179 Extensive lymphangiosarcoma complicating lymphoedema.

Index